ICE CREAM BOOK

100 Best and Delicious Ice Cream Recipes

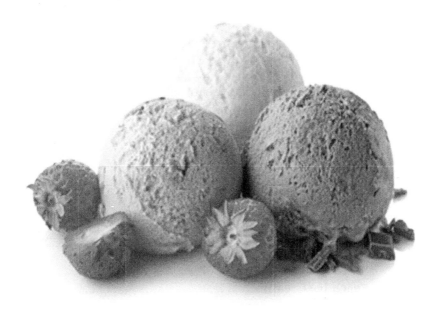

Inna Volia

TABLE OF CONTENTS

INTRODUCTION

Dear reader! Thank you very much for buying this book of ice cream recipes.

There is no one definition of or recipe for ice cream. However, ice cream typically contains cream (hence, ice cream). Ice cream is one of the most favorite desserts for both children and adults; and the best way to cool off on a hot summer day! Recipes of this dessert were cherished and passed throughout generations of families. While ice cream is served across the continents, it was not until the invention of refrigeration that it became famous as a dessert.

This book contains 100 homemade ice cream recipes which means, you can now enjoy frozen treats, and serve your kids too, without being worried about those scary chemicals in store-bought ice cream. You are on a great ice cream journey, and you will never look back to that store-bought stuff! The ingredients listed in this book are not obligatory, and you can replace some of them with your favorites not being afraid of spoiling the dish.

Now that you know what we have to offer to you through this great cookbook, will you make the best decision of your life? So, get it today and get ready to have your dessert world changed and discover the rich, fantastic taste of homemade ice cream. And don't feel bad when you eat the whole batch...I know you'll want to! Have a lot of fun this summer!

Basics of Ice cream

There are hundreds of ice cream recipes out there. Each one has its unique name, ingredient, measurement, preparation duration and country of origin. But beyond these differences, all ice cream recipes have something in common called a base. *A base* is the foundation of ice cream. It is a process of mixing ingredients which will, later on, turn into tasty and sumptuous looking ice creams.

There are four kinds of bases unique to ice cream recipes.

1. The Custard Base

It is easy and very similar to making pudding or custard. It involves mixing egg yolk with sugar and cream.

2. The Egg Free Base

The base is prepared without the use of egg. It is a mixture of cream, milk, and cheese. It uses cornstarch as a thickener. The base gives the ice cream a soft and silky outlook.

3. Philadelphia- Style Base

It is similar to the egg-free base because it also does not utilize eggs. The foundation is a combination of sugar, cream, and flavoring. To help the sugar dissolve, we can subject the base for cooking or heating though it is not necessary. A weakness of this base is that it does not have a substantial nutritional value and fat content like the custard base. However, the addition of cream tries to boost the fat content of this base.

4. No Churn Base.

This is the most distinct of the four bases. It is only one that does require cooking unlike the other three. We also do not need an ice cream maker. The ingredients needed to make this base are a large mixture amount of cream and sweetened condensed milk (very high in fat content).

The condensed milk functions as the thick base while the cream is added to it to give a smooth and glossy texture. Ice

Types of Ice creams

1. Gelato

. It is a famous Italian frozen dessert made from fresh cow's milk, cream, and sugar, with berries, nuts, chocolate, and fresh fruits. Gelato incorporates less air than ice cream, creating denser, more flavorful results.

2. Sorbet

Sorbet is a frozen dessert made from sugar syrup and fruit juice. It is a quick and straightforward dessert without the use of dairy products. Typically, sorbets do not include any dairy, though this isn't a hard and fast rule. They are incredibly simple to produce. You will find that removing sorbet from the freezer 8–10 minutes before serving aids in scooping; as sorbets freeze harder than ice creams or gelato do because they contain no fat ingredients.

3. Sherbets

Sherbets are similar to sorbets in that they contain few ingredients. The difference is that Sherbets tend to contain milk or cream. Fresh, ripe fruits are the stars here, and it's as simple as puréeing all ingredients together in a blender or food processor and freezing in an ice cream machine. Like sorbet, it is a good idea to remove sherbet from the freezer a few minutes before serving for best results.

4. Frozen Yogurt

Frozen delights composed of—you guessed it—yogurt. Cream and milk are also common ingredients in this variety of dessert. Both Greek yogurt and standard yogurts are excellent bases and can be used interchangeably if desired. In a pinch, or as an added twist, sour cream can be substituted for part (or all, if desired) of the yogurt for either variety. This will, of course, result in a sourer end product, but is quite refreshing when paired with a variety of fruits, such as blueberries.

5. Granita

It is a Sicilian dessert with crushed fruit ice and sugar. It is a variety of sorbets but has a more dense structure. Perfect idea for summer parties and picnics! You can also cook it with alcohol to make a cocktail! It requires nothing more than a fork and a freezer to obtain quality results.

Why Homemade Ice Creams?

Fresh Ingredients- When you make ice creams at home, you use fresh ingredients without adding any preservatives and colors.

Sharp Brain & Mental focus - Processed commercial ice cream adversely affects our brain's cognitive functionality, responsiveness, and memory. Homemade ice cream is a healthy alternative to improve your brain health.

Young Skin- Added with the power of natural fruit and spices, homemade ice cream helps you to keep your skin look vibrant and refreshingly youthful. Processed commercial ice cream makes our skin wrinkled and dull through a process known as "glycation"; which damages the elastic property of the skin and makes it look saggy.

Weight Control- Healthy homemade ice cream provides you with the power to keep your weight in check and maintain your fit lifestyle.

Satiety value- Homemade ice cream makes you feel full by keeping control over your appetite level. It helps you minimize overall food intake and makes way for a healthy lifestyle.

The Ingredients

1. CREAM

There are Different versions of cream contain different fat contents. That means, when you want it richer, you need to increase the fat content in your cream, and vice versa. The benefit of the added fat is that heavier cream holds its peak longer.

2. MILK

Milk along with cream makes your ice cream flavorful and creamy. Popular milk varieties are full-fat milk, condensed milk, coconut milk, soymilk, and half-and-half. Experiments with richer or lighter milk will alter your results only slightly.

3. EGGS

The richness of your ice cream custard base is derived from protein-rich egg yolks. Rich egg custard is a harmonious blend of milk, cream and sugar thickened slowly over gentle heat. Choose extra-large organic eggs, which are the standard size for all the recipes in this book. Using medium or jumbo eggs won't harm a recipe much, especially if it calls for only one egg. The need to stick to large eggs is just an issue when you begin to multiply a recipe by 10 or 20.

4. SUGAR AND SWEETENERS

Organic granulated sugar, unless otherwise noted in recipes where confectioners' sugar is called for. It works as a sweet component to your homemade ice cream.

5. SALT

Salt is the magical mineral that enhances flavor, which is why salt is an ingredient in nearly every recipe of this book. In most cases, it is not intended to add saltiness. Just a pinch brings out the natural flavors of the dish. Left out, the recipes will seem bland.

6. SWEETENED CONDENSED MILK

It is used, however, in the gelato chapter to enrich the ice cream bases. As stated earlier, sweetened condensed milk is used as a replacement for the classic ice cream custard.

7. FRUIT AND NUTS.

Fruit is a healthy addition to any ice cream recipe; in fact, it represents the real asset to various ices. You get an opportunity to taste varietals, comparing texture, sweetness, flavor, and color. Examples are mango, strawberries, blueberries, cinnamon, raisin, peach and pineapple.

8. EXTRACTS

For example, vanilla, peppermint, almond, and maple flavorings

9. CHOCOLATE

For bolder results, explore the spectrum of higher cacao percentages.

10. ALCOHOL

The right amount of alcohol and the finished dessert is rendered complex and luscious; too much and the mixture will not correctly set and will remain slushy and unappealing.

11. UNFLAVORED GELATIN

The second option for thickener is gelatin. It's dairy-free but not vegetarian.

Essential Tools to Make Ice Cream at Home

- **FREEZER BOWLS/CONTAINERS**

This is to store your ice cream mixtures. Choose bowls and containers that have a high surface area as they allow the mixture to settle down faster and make it richer. Many containers or bowls come with covers, choose the one with covers as they prevent air circulation.

- **FORKS AND WHISKS**

A fork is used for blending, stirring and prodding an ice cream mixture, while whisks are used to whisk egg yolks, creams, etc.

- **FINE-MESH STRAINER**

The texture is very important, and that is why many ice cream mixtures need to be passed through the sieve to remove hard ingredients and make the texture smooth.

- **SCOOPER**

To scoop and serve ice cream

- **TIMERS**

- **A WOODEN SPOON (OPTIONAL)**

For testing the progress of the base as it thickens.

- **A BLENDER OR FOOD PROCESSOR**

For grinding nuts and puréeing fruits and other mixtures

ICE CREAM RECIPES

CLASSIC ICE CREAM TREATS

1) Classic Vanilla Ice Cream

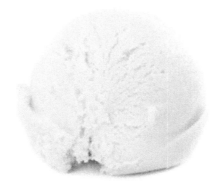

Servings: 8
Total Prep time: 4 hours

Ingredients:
- 4 cups half-and-half,
- 1/2 cup heavy cream,
- 3/4 cups sugar
- 2 tsp vanilla extract
- Pinch of salt

Directions:
1. Whisk all ingredients together until all well mixed and some air has been incorporated into the mix.
2. Pour the mix into a shallow pan and place the pan in the freezer.

3. After 30 minutes, open the freezer and stir the mixture vigorously with a spatula or spoon.
4. Place the pan back in the freezer.
5. Continue to do this every 30 minutes for the next three hours and your ice cream should be ready to eat.
6. Enjoy.

2) Chocolate Ice Cream

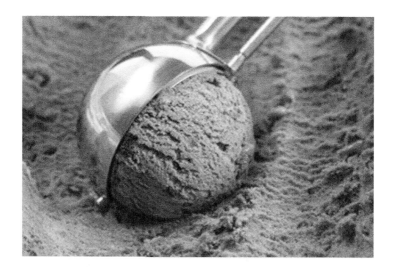

Servings: 8
Total Prep time: 1 hour

Ingredients:
- 14oz can of sweetened condensed milk
- 2 cups heavy cream
- 1/2 cup cocoa powder
- 1 tsp vanilla extract
- Pinch salt

Directions:
1. Whisk together the milk, cocoa powder, vanilla, and salt until they are all combined.
2. In a different bowl whisk the cream until firm peaks appearing in around two minutes.
3. Fold one cup of the whipped cream into the first mixture until it is thoroughly combined.
4. Pour this mix back into the rest of the whipped cream and fold until it is all mixed.

5. Pour this mix into a shallow pan and put it in the freezer and leave it in the freezer for two to three hours.
6. When it is frozen, scoop it into bowls and enjoy.

3) Nutty Ice Cream

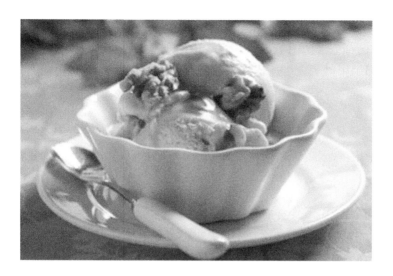

Servings: 16
Total Prep time: 2 hours and 10 minutes
Cook time: 20 minutes

Ingredients:
- 1 tablespoon butter
- 1 cup brown sugar
- 1/3 cup pecans, chopped
- 2 eggs, whisked
- 1 teaspoon vanilla extract
- 1 and ½ cups half and half
- ½ cup heavy cream

Directions:
1. Heat up a pan over medium heat, add pecans, stir and toast for 5 minutes.
2. In another pan, mix sugar with half and half, stir and bring to a boil over medium-high heat.
3. Take off heat and mix with eggs and butter.

4. Return this to heat, stir and cook until it thickens.
5. Take off the heat again, add toasted pecans, heavy cream, and vanilla, stir, transfer to an ice cream maker, process and freeze for 2 hours before serving.
6. Enjoy!

4) Peanut Butter Ice Cream

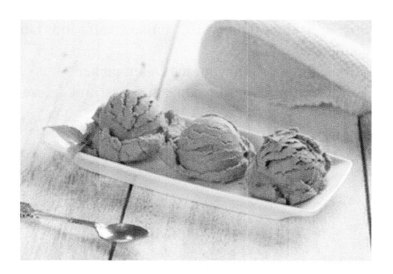

Servings: 8
Total Prep time: 3hours
Cook time: 5 minutes

Ingredients:
- 3 eggs
- ½ cup half and half
- ¼ cup sugar
- ¾ cup canned condensed milk
- 2 teaspoons vanilla extract
- 1 cup whole milk
- ¾ cup peanut butter
- 12 mini peanut butter cups, chopped

Directions:
1. In a bowl beat with your mixer eggs and sugar.
2. Heat up a pan with whole milk over medium heat and then pour it over the eggs.

3. Stir this mix and transfer it to a pan. Heat up over low heat for 3 minutes, take off heat and add peanut butter.
4. Stir and then mix with vanilla, half and half and condensed milk.
5. Stir again; pour into your ice cream maker.
6. Fold in peanut butter cups, process and freeze for 3 hours.
7. Enjoy!

5) Cinnamon Ice Cream

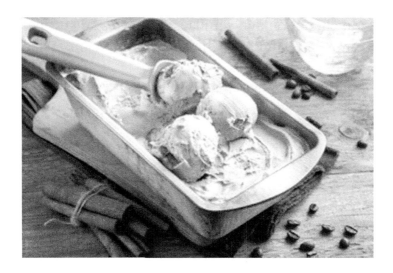

Servings: 8
Total Prep time: 2 hours
Cook time: 15 minutes

Ingredients:
- 1 cup heavy cream
- 1 cup white sugar
- 2 eggs, whisked
- 2 teaspoons cinnamon, ground
- 1 teaspoon vanilla extract
- 1 and ½ cups half and half

Directions:
1. Put half and half in a pot and heat up over medium heat.
2. Add sugar, stir, bring to a simmer and take off heat.
3. Add half of the eggs and stir continuously add the rest of the eggs, stir and heat up the mix again over medium heat.

4. Add heavy cream, stir, cook until it thickens and take off the heat again.
5. Add cinnamon and vanilla, stir, leave aside to cool down completely and pour into an ice cream maker and process.
6. Freeze according to instructions and serve.
7. Enjoy!

6) Coconut Ice Cream

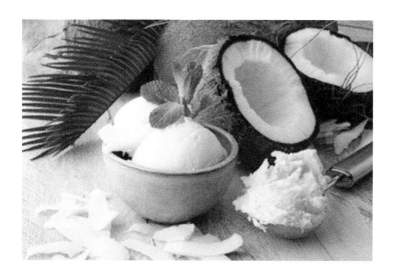

Servings: 6
Total Prep time: 30 minutes

Ingredients:

- 14 ounces canned cream of coconut
- 1 cup milk
- 1 and ½ cup coconut, sweet and flaked
- 1 and ½ cups heavy cream

Directions:

1. In your food processor, mix cream of coconut with milk and pulse well.
2. Add cream and coconut, blend again, transfer to your ice cream maker, process according to instructions and freeze for at least 30 minutes.
3. Enjoy!

7) Green Tea Ice Cream

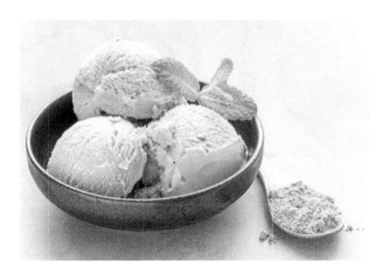

Servings: 4
Total Prep time: 6 hours and 5 minutes

Ingredients:
- 4 tablespoons canned sweetened condensed milk
- 1 cup heavy cream
- 3 tablespoons hot water
- 4 and ½ teaspoons green tea powder

Directions:
1. In a bowl, mix green tea powder with hot water, stir well and leave aside until it's cold.
2. Add condensed milk and stir again thoroughly.
3. Add heavy cream, stir, pour into a container and keep in the freezer for 6 hours before serving.
4. Enjoy!

8) Beer Ice Cream

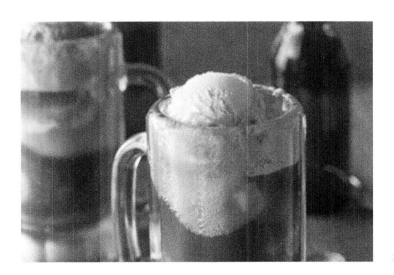

Servings: 8
Total Prep time: 5 hours
Cook time: 5 minutes

Ingredients:
- 6 egg yolks, whisked
- 2 cups heavy whipping cream
- 1 vanilla bean, seeds scraped
- 1 and ½ cups whole milk
- 1 cup sugar
- 12 ounces Irish beer

Directions:
1. Put cream in a pot and heat up over medium heat.
2. Add milk and sugar, stir well for 2 minutes and take off heat.
3. Add vanilla seeds and stir.
4. Add egg yolks, stir, heat up again and cook for 3 minutes more.

5. Transfer this to a bowl and keep in the fridge for 2 hours.
6. Heat up the beer in a pot, bring to a simmer and reduce to half.
7. Keep this in the fridge for 2 hours as well.
8. Combine cream mix with beer, stir well, transfer to an ice cream maker, then process according to instructions and freeze for at least 1 hour.
9. Enjoy!

9) Eggnog Ice Cream

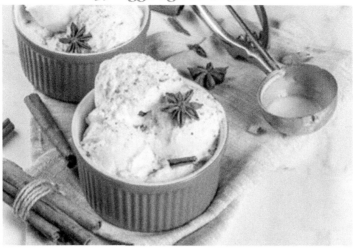

Servings: 10
Total Prep time: 2 hours

Ingredients:
- 10 ounces canned and sweetened condensed milk
- 2 cups eggnog
- 2 cups heavy cream
- 1 teaspoon vanilla extract

Directions:
1. In a bowl, combine all ingredients and whisk well.
2. Pour this into your ice cream maker, process according to instructions and freeze for at least 2 hours.
3. Enjoy!

10)   Snow Ice Cream

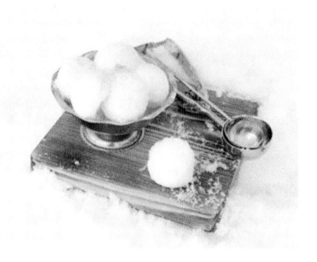

Servings: 8
Total Prep time: 5 minutes

Ingredients:
- 1 tablespoon vanilla extract
- 2 cups milk
- 1 cup sugar
- 1-gallon snow

Directions:
1. Put 1-gallon snow in a bowl, add milk, sugar, and vanilla, stir and serve right away!
2. Enjoy!

11) Cake Mix Ice Cream

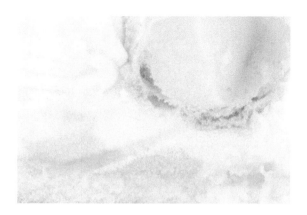

Servings: 6
Total Prep time: 2 hours
Cook time: 5 minutes

Ingredients:

- 2 egg yolks, whisked
- ½ cup white sugar
- 1 cup milk
- 2 cups heavy cream
- 1 teaspoon vanilla extract
- ¾ cup sifted cake mix

Directions:

1. Put the milk in a pan and heat up over medium-low heat.
2. Add the rest of the ingredients and stir well for about 5 minutes and take off from the heat.
3. Transfer to a container and keep in a fridge until its cold.
4. Transfer ice cream mix to an ice cream maker, process and freeze for 2 hours.
5. Enjoy!

12) Tropical Ice Cream

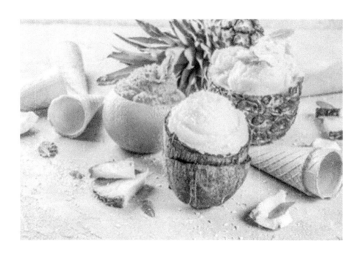

Servings: 6
Total Prep time: 50 minutes

Ingredients:
- 1 banana, peeled and sliced
- 1/3 cup walnuts, chopped
- 1/3 cup coconut, flaked
- 2 cups heavy cream
- 1 and ½ cups milk
- 2/3 cup pineapple and orange juice
- ¾ cup sugar

Directions:
1. In a large bowl, mix banana with cream, milk, sugar and pineapple and orange juice mix.
2. Stir well, pour into your ice cream maker, process and freeze for 45 minutes.
3. Add walnuts and coconut, fold them in gently and freeze for 5 minutes more.
4. Enjoy!

13)   Creamy Chocolate Ice Cream

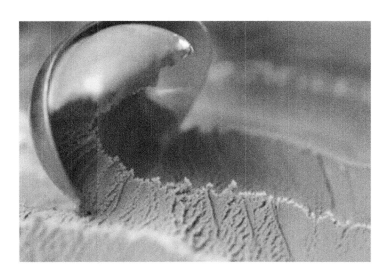

Servings: 12
Total Prep time: 6 hours

Ingredients:
- 2/3 cup chocolate syrup
- 2 cups heavy cream
- 14 ounces canned condensed milk

Directions:
1. In a bowl, mix heavy cream with condensed milk and chocolate syrup and stir well to combine.
2. Pour this into a loaf pan, spread, introduce in your freezer for 6 hours and then serve.
3. Enjoy!

14)   Choco Pecan Ice Cream

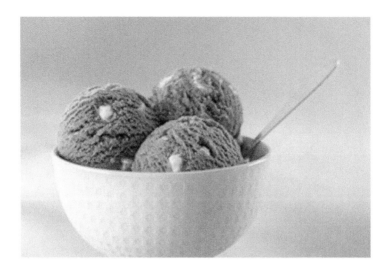

Servings: 7
Total Prep time: 1 hour
Cook time: 5 minutes

Ingredients:
- 1 tablespoon vanilla extract
- ½ cup pecans, chopped
- 2 cups heavy cream
- 14 ounces canned and sweetened condensed milk
- ½ cup cocoa powder
- 1 cup mini marshmallows
- 1 cup light cream

Directions:
1. Heat up a pan over medium-low heat, add cocoa powder and condensed milk, stir well, cook for 5 minutes, and take off heat and leave aside to cool down.
2. Add light cream, heavy cream and vanilla extract, stir well again and leave aside to cool down completely.

3. Transfer this to your ice cream machine and freeze according to directions for 30 minutes.
4. Add marshmallows and nuts, stir and freeze for 30 minutes more.
5. Enjoy!

15)   Coconut Cacao Ice Cream

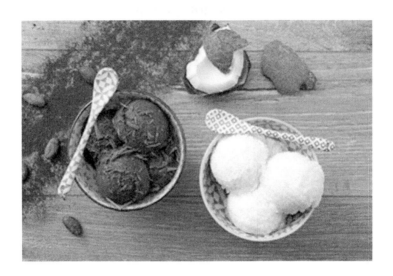

Servings: 6
Total Prep time: 1 hour

Ingredients:

- 1 1/2 cups coconut milk
- 1/2 cup heavy cream
- 1/2 tsp vanilla
- 2 Tbsp sugar,
- Pinch of salt
- Coconut flakes (As much as you want)
- Cacao nibs (As much as you want)

Directions:

1. Combine the milk, cream, vanilla, sugar, and salt.
2. Whisk these ingredients together.
3. Once incorporated, add the coconut flakes and cacao nibs to the mix and place in the small bag.
4. Shake the mix and freeze for 1 hour.
5. Enjoy.

16)   Mint Choc Oreo Ice Cream

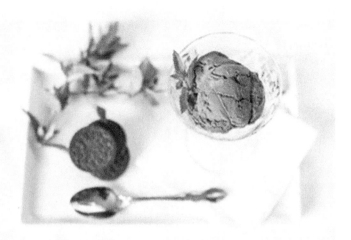

Servings: 5
Total Prep time: 1 hour

Ingredients:
- 1 cup whipping cream
- 2 Tbsp sugar
- 1/4 tsp peppermint extract
- 4 drops green food coloring (optional)
- 5 Oreos

Directions:
1. Mix the whipping cream, sugar, and peppermint and add to the smaller bag.
2. You can add the food coloring to the mix if you want the green tint that looks like the store bought ice cream.
3. Shake the mix and then transfer to a bowl.
4. Crush the Oreos and stir them into the ice cream.
5. Freeze for an hour.
6. Enjoy.

17)Cinnamon Coconut Ice Cream

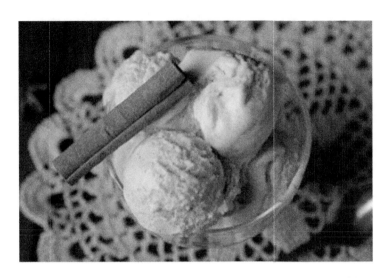

Servings: 6
Total Prep time: 1 hour

Ingredients:

- 2 cans coconut milk (At room temperature)
- 1/4 cup honey
- 3 egg yolks
- 2 tsp cinnamon

Directions:

1. Separate 3 eggs and use the yolks for the ice cream.
2. Add the honey and cinnamon to the egg yolks and whisk together.
3. Add the coconut milk and whisk together.
4. Put the mixture into the smaller bag.
5. Shake the mix and enjoy immediately or freeze for later.
6. Enjoy.

18) Rich and Delicious Chocolate Ice Cream

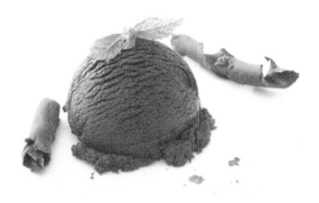

Servings: 8
Total Prep time: 4 hours
Cook time: 10 minutes

Ingredients:
- 3 egg yolks, whisked
- ¾ cup sugar
- 1 cup milk
- 2 ounces semisweet chocolate, chopped
- 2 tablespoons cocoa powder
- A pinch of salt
- 1 teaspoon vanilla extract
- 2 cup heavy cream

Directions:
1. Put milk in a pot and heat up over medium heat. Add salt, cocoa powder and sugar, stir and bring to a simmer.

2. In a bowl, mix egg yolks with ½ cup milk and stir. Add this to the pot, stir until it thickens and take off heat.
3. Add chocolate, stir and keep in the fridge for 2 hours.
4. Add vanilla and cream stir transfer to your ice cream maker, then process according to instructions and freeze for 2 hours.
5. Enjoy!

19)   Delectable fruity Ice Cream

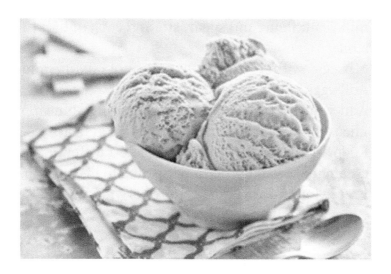

Servings: 28
Total Prep time: 1 hour
Cook time: 10 minutes

Ingredients:

- 1-quart chocolate milk
- 1 tablespoon vanilla extract
- 2 cups sugar
- 3 tablespoons flour
- A pinch of salt
- 1-quart milk
- 12 ounces canned evaporated milk
- 20 ounces chopped strawberries
- 2 bananas, peeled and chopped
- 15 ounces canned crushed pineapple and juice
- 6 eggs whisked

Directions:

1. Heat up a pan over medium heat, add milk, evaporated milk, salt, flour, and sugar, stir and cook until it thickens a bit.
2. Mix eggs with 1 tablespoon of this hot mixture and stir.
3. Add eggs to the pan and stir very well.
4. Add strawberries, vanilla, chocolate milk, pineapple and juice, and bananas, stir well and take off heat.
5. Keep in the fridge until it's cold, transfer to your ice cream maker and process according to instructions.
6. Freeze for at least 1 hour before serving.
7. Enjoy!

20)   Vibrant Strawberry Ice Cream

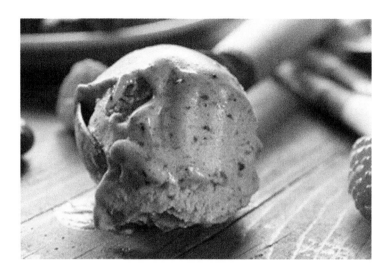

Servings: 6
Total Prep time: 1 hour and 10 minutes
Cook time: 10 minutes

Ingredients:
- 1 and ½ cups heavy cream
- 1-quart strawberries halved
- 3 egg yolks
- ¾ cup sugar
- 3 tablespoons corn syrup

Directions:
1. Put strawberries in your blender, pulse well, transfer to a bowl and leave aside for now.
2. Heat up a pan over medium heat, add 1 and ¼ cups cream, stir and bring to a gentle simmer.
3. Meanwhile, in a bowl, mix the rest of the cream with egg yolks, corn syrup, and sugar and stir well.

41

4. Pour this into the pan stirring often and heat up for 5 minutes more.
5. Strain this mix, add strawberries puree, whisk well and keep in the fridge until it's cold.
6. Transfer this to your ice cream maker, process and freeze for 1 hour.
7. Enjoy!

21)   Chocolate Chip Ice Cream

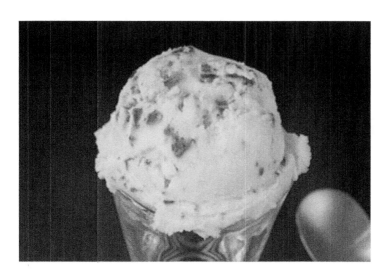

Servings: 5
Total Prep time: 1 hour 10 minutes

Ingredients:
- 1 cup milk
- 3 Tbsp sugar
- 3 drops almond extract
- 2 Tbsp chocolate chips

Directions:

1. Mix the milk, sugar, almond extract, and chocolate chips and add to the small bag.
2. Shake the mix and freeze
3. Enjoy.

22)   Berry Ice Cream

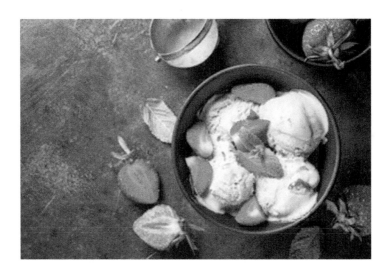

Servings: 6
Total Prep time: 1 hour

Ingredients:
- 1 cup half-and-half
- 1/3 cup powdered sugar
- 1/4 cup frozen berries

Directions:
1. Mix the half-and-half and powdered sugar until the powdered sugar is dissolved.
2. Add the berries to the mix and place in the smaller bag. Shake the mix and freeze.
3. Enjoy.

23)   Strawberry Ice Cream

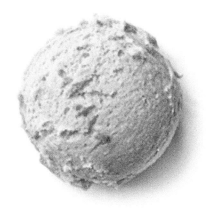

Servings: 9
Total Prep time: 5 hours

Ingredients:
- 1 pound frozen strawberries
- 2 cups heavy cream
- 14oz sweetened condensed milk
- 1 tsp vanilla extract
- Pinch of salt

Directions:
1. Allow the strawberries to rise in temperature slightly by taking them out of the freezer ten minutes before starting this recipe.
2. Use a blender/food processor to cut the strawberries into small chunks.
3. Mix the milk, vanilla, salt, and strawberry chunks in a bowl.
4. In a separate bowl, whisk up the cream, either by hand or with an electric mixer until firm peaks form.

5. Fold a cup of the cream into the strawberry mixture and then pour this mixture back into the whipped cream.
6. Blend the mixtures until thoroughly mixed.
7. Pour the mixture into a shallow pan, or loaf tin, and place it in the freezer.
8. Let it sit in the freezer for 4-5 hours before scooping into bowls and enjoying.

24)   Peach Ice Cream

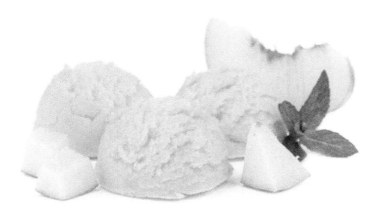

Servings: 30
Total Prep time: 1 hour and 10 minutes

Ingredients:
- ½ cup white sugar
- 1 pint half and half
- 2 and ½ pounds peaches, pitted, peeled and chopped
- 12 ounces canned evaporated milk
- 2 cups whole milk
- 1 teaspoon vanilla extract
- 14 ounces canned condensed milk

Directions:
1. Put peaches in your blender and pulse well.
2. Add half and half and sugar and blend again.
3. Put this into a bowl and combine with condensed milk, vanilla and evaporated milk.
4. Pour this into a container, add whole milk, stir gently and keep in the freezer for 1 hour before you serve it.
5. Enjoy!

25)   Blueberry Ice Cream

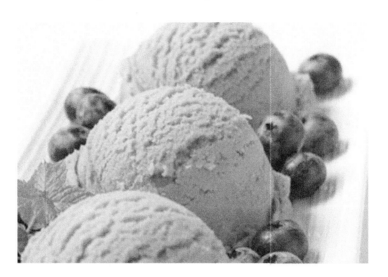

Servings: 15
Total Prep time: 20 minutes + inactive time

Ingredients:

- 2 cups fresh blueberries
- 1 cup whipping cream
- 4 whole eggs
- 1 cup full-fat milk
- 1 cup filtered water
- ½ cup caster sugar
- 1 teaspoon vanilla paste
- 1 pinches salt

Directions:

1. In a saucepan, whisk the water, milk, eggs, sugar, and salt.
2. Heat the mixture over medium-high heat and bring to a gentle bubble.
3. Strain into a full bowl and chill.

4. Whisk in the vanilla, whipping cream and fresh blueberries.
5. Cover the ice cream mix and freeze for 4-6 hours, stirring after each hour to prevent ice crystal formation.
6. Serve and enjoy.

LOW CARB & LOW SUGAR ICE CREAMS

26)   Irish ice cream

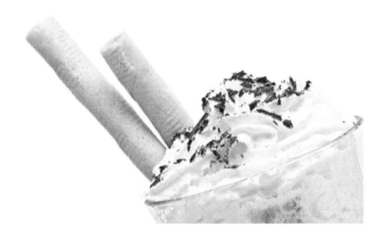

Servings: 6
Total Prep time: 20 minutes

Ingredients:
- 300ml double cream
- 100ml Irish cream syrup
- 4 eggs
- 4 teaspoons chocolate syrup
- 3 teaspoons stevia

Directions:
1. Whisk stevia with double cream with a hand whisk.
2. Pre-heat a saucepan over medium-low heat; transfer whisked cream.

3. Add Irish cream syrup and chocolate syrup, mix thoroughly.
4. Bring the mixture to a boil stirring constantly.
5. Whisk eggs in a bowl, add one-third of the egg mixture to the saucepan, mix well, and then add the remaining mass.
6. Chill the mixture in the ice water for 10 minutes.
7. Blend the chilled mixture with an electrical blender.
8. Transfer to a container and freeze for 10-12 hours.

27)   Berry ice cream

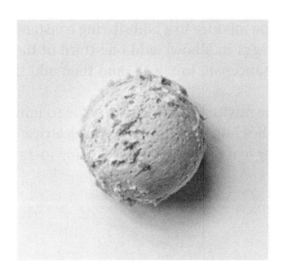

Servings: 2
Total Prep time: 10 Hours 35 minutes

Ingredients:
- 250g double cream
- 70g sugar
- 50g currant
- 50g strawberries
- 4 eggs

Directions:
1. Pre-heat a saucepan over medium heat and add double cream. Heat it for 5-10 minutes until you get a liquid structure.
2. Separate egg whites from yolks; whisk the egg yolks with sugar thoroughly until the sugar dissolves.
3. Stir whisked eggs in the double cream and mix well. Remove from heat and cool for 25-30 minutes.

4. Blend strawberries and currants with an electrical blender, strain through the sieve.
5. Add fruit to the cooled mixture, mix thoroughly.
6. Transfer the mixture to a container and freeze for overnight.

28)   Creamy ice cream

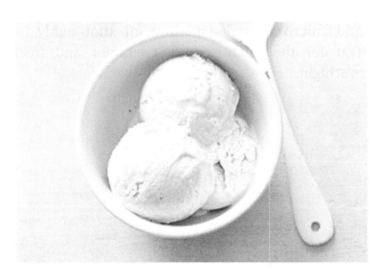

Servings: 3
Total Prep time: 10 hours 25 minutes

Ingredients:
- 100ml double cream
- 3 eggs
- 3 teaspoons stevia extract
- 1 teaspoon vanilla extract

Directions:
1. Separate egg whites from yolks and whisk the yolks.
2. Pre-heat a saucepan over low heat, pour double cream.
3. Add stevia and vanilla extract, heat for 5-6 minutes stirring constantly.
4. Remove the saucepan from the heat every 2 minutes so as not to bring the mixture to a simmer.
5. Slowly stir in the whisked yolks, mix well.
6. Cool the mixture in the fridge for 10 minutes.

7. Blend it with an electric blender for 5 minutes, transfer to a container.
8. Put the mixture in the freezer for 10 hours.
9. Enjoy.

29)   Coffee ice cream

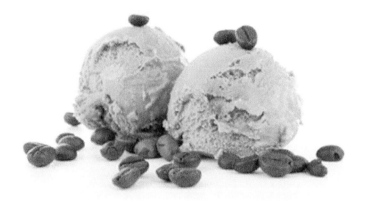

Servings: 5
Total Prep time: 7 hours 15 minutes

Ingredients:
- 200ml double cream
- 100ml milk
- 5g instant coffee
- 5 teaspoons stevia extract
- 1 teaspoon vanilla extract

Directions:
1. Combine double cream and milk in the bowl, whisk them to firm peaks.
2. Combine instant coffee with ½ teaspoon water and add to whisked mixture.
3. Add stevia and vanilla extract and mix with an electric blender for 10 minutes until you get a homogenous structure.
4. Transfer the mixture to a container and put it in the freezer for 7 hours.

30)   Ricotta ice cream

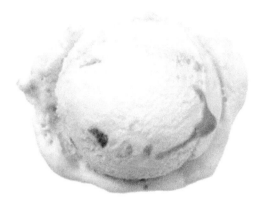

Servings: 3
Total Prep time: 5 hours 25 minutes

Ingredients:
- 100ml whipping cream
- 50ml coconut milk
- 50g ricotta cheese (chopped)
- 50g sugar
- 3 teaspoons stevia
- 1 teaspoon vanilla extract

Directions:
1. Whisk whipping cream in a bowl to get soft peaks.
2. Pour coconut milk into the bowl, mix well.
3. Add sugar and combine thoroughly until the sugar dissolves.
4. Add ricotta cheese to the mixture.
5. Blend it with an electrical blender.
6. Add stevia and vanilla extract, stir with a hand whisk.

7. Put the mixture in the freezer for 15-20 minutes, stir again.
8. Transfer the mixture to a container and freeze for 5 more hours.

31) Chocolate ice cream

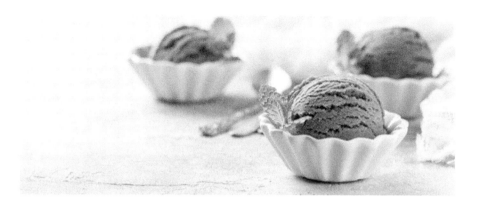

Servings: 6
Total Prep time: 5 hours

Ingredients:
- 300ml double cream
- 100ml coconut milk
- 30g cocoa powder
- 4 eggs
- 2 teaspoons stevia
- 1 teaspoon vanilla extract

Directions:
1. Pre-heat a saucepan over medium-low heat.
2. Beat double cream and combine with coconut milk.
3. Mix thoroughly.
4. Transfer the mixture to the saucepan and add cocoa powder and vanilla extract mix well.
5. Freeze for 4 hours.

32)   Lemon Ice-Cream

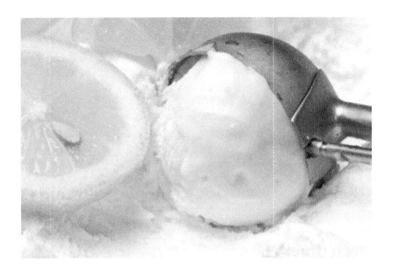

Servings: 8
Total Prep time: 1 hour 15 minutes

Ingredients:
- ¾ cup of heavy cream
- 2/3 cup lemon juice
- 1 ½ teaspoons vanilla extract
- ¼ teaspoon lemon zest
- 3 drops yellow food coloring
- 2 tablespoons glycerin
- A pinch of sea salt
- 3 eggs
- 2 tablespoons butter
- Stevia to taste
- 3 cups full cream milk

Directions:

1. Blend in a mixing bowl milk, lemon juice, eggs, salt, cream, blending until smooth.
2. Pour mixture into a saucepan and bring to a boil over medium-high heat on top of the stove.
3. When bubbles begin to appear to remove the mix from heat and stir in remaining ingredients.
4. Allow mix to cool at room temperature.
5. Add to an ice-cream maker, churn according to directions.
6. Freeze, scoop and enjoy this refreshing sweet treat!

33)   Cherry Chocolate Chip Ice-Cream

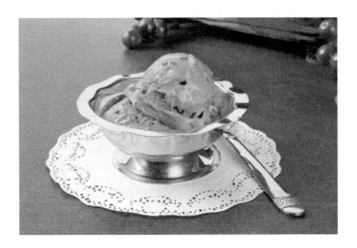

Servings: 8
Total Prep time: 3 hours

Ingredients:
- 1 tablespoon of scraped vanilla bean
- 10 ounces cherries, pitted
- 13.5 ounces coconut milk
- 1 tablespoon glycerin
- ½ cup unsweetened chocolate chips
- Erythritol to taste

Directions:
1. Take 3 ounces of cherries and set them aside.
2. Blend the remaining cherries, vanilla, milk, and sweetener.
3. Mix cherries in by hand.
4. Pour into ice-cream maker and churn until set.
5. Just before you turn it off add in the chocolate chips and run it for an additional minute.
6. Freeze, scoop and enjoy!

34)   Strawberry Ice-Cream

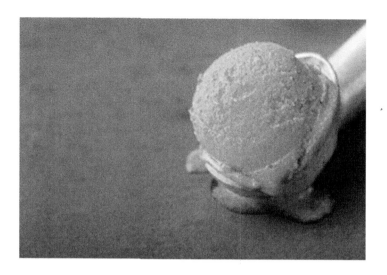

Servings: 8
Total Prep time: 3 hours

Ingredients:
- 1 cup of heavy cream
- 3 cups of full cream milk
- 3 cups of fresh sliced strawberries
- 1 teaspoon vanilla extract
- 2/3 cup cottage cheese
- Stevia to taste
- Dash of sea salt
- ½ teaspoon Guar gum

Directions:
1. Blend all your ingredients until they are smooth.
2. Pour into your ice-cream maker and churn until you reach desired consistency.
3. Freeze, scoop and enjoy!

35)   Peaches & Cream Ice-Cream

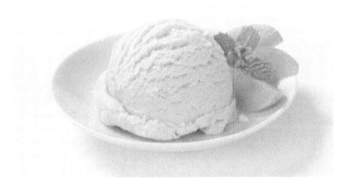

Servings: 8
Total Prep time: 12 hours 10 minutes

Ingredients:
- 3 drops of Orange food coloring
- 2 cups heavy cream
- 3 large peaches
- Erythritol to taste
- ½ cup water
- 1 ½ cups half and half

Directions:
1. Peel and dice your peaches, then set aside. Puree one peach with water and set aside.
2. Whisk sweetener, cream, peach puree, and food coloring together with the half and half.
3. Pour the mixture into your ice cream maker and churn according to the directions.

4. When your ice-cream begins to firm up, add in the chopped peaches.
5. Freeze the mix overnight.

*** To keep the ice cream soft, add in Xanthan gum.

36)   Blueberry Pancake Ice-Cream

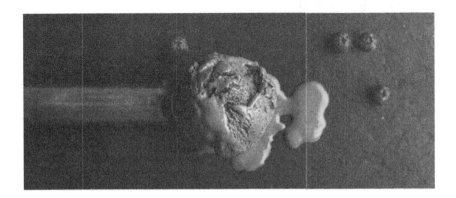

Servings: 8
Total Prep time: 12 hours

Ingredients:
- 1 cup heavy cream
- 1 teaspoon of red wine vinegar
- 1 1/8 cup of buttermilk
- 1 ½ tablespoon of glycerin
- Pinch of sea salt
- Stevia to taste

For Puree:
- ½ lb of blueberries
- 2 tablespoons of lime juice, fresh
- 1/8 teaspoon of nutmeg, ground
- 1/8 teaspoon of almond extract
- 1/8 teaspoon of cinnamon, ground
- Stevia to taste
- ¼ teaspoon vanilla extract
- 1 tablespoon water

Directions:

1. In a small saucepan add in lime juice, water, blueberries, and spices.
2. Heat mixture over low heat until softened.
3. Using a wooden spoon mash the mix.
4. Puree the mix using an immersion blender. Add in the vanilla, almond extract, and Stevia.
5. Cook mix on simmer until it develops a syrupy consistency. Add in a splash of water if needed. Remove mix from heat and allow cooling at room temperature.
6. Add the mix to your ice cream maker and churn until set.
7. Freeze, scoop and serve your yummy keto sweet treat!

37) Watermelon Frozen Puree

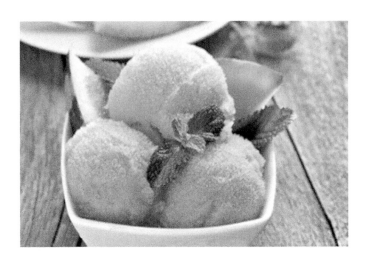

Servings: 8
Total Prep time: 12 hours

Ingredients:
- 8 cups of diced watermelon
- 2 cups of coconut milk
- 2 teaspoons of lemon juice, fresh
- Liquid Stevia to taste

Directions:
1. Freeze your watermelon overnight.
2. Placed the diced watermelon in your food processor and began to mix it at low speed.
3. When it becomes puree-like, add in the coconut milk along with the rest of the ingredients.
4. Continue to blend and pause every once and a while to scrap the sides of the bowl.
5. Eventually, air will be incorporated into the fruit, and it will gain a sherbet-like consistency to it.
6. Scoop and serve immediately.

38)   Strawberry Swirl Ice Cream

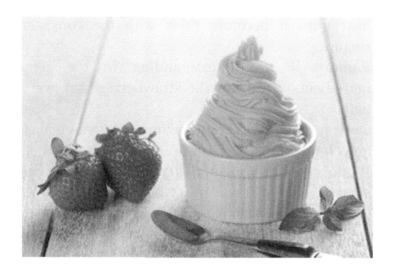

Servings: 8
Total Prep time: 4 hours

Ingredients:
- 2 tablespoons of glycerin
- 1 ¼ cups heavy whipping cream
- 3 egg yolks
- 4 ounces cream cheese
- 1 cup full cream milk
- 1 cup strawberries, frozen
- ½ teaspoon vanilla extract
- ½ teaspoon Xanthan gum
- Stevia to taste

Directions:
1. Whisk your egg yolks until they are smooth, along with sweetener. In a saucepan, mix the milk and cream.
2. Bring to a boil.

3. Pour over egg yolks while you whisk mix. Return the combination to the saucepan and cook over medium heat until it becomes thick with the consistency of custard.
4. Remove it from heat adding in the remaining ingredients except for the strawberries, set over an ice bath.
5. Once it has cooled pour mixture into ice cream maker and churn.
6. While you are churning mash the strawberries with some powdered Stevia or Erythritol.
7. Make sure the mash is a nice goop-like mixture.
8. Add in water if needed.
9. Just before you turn off the ice cream maker pour in the strawberries and allow it to churn for another few minutes.
10. Remove and freeze.

39) Double Chocolate Delight Ice cream

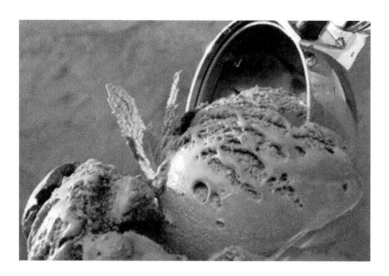

Servings: 8
Total Prep time: 3 hours

Ingredients:
- ½ cup cocoa powder
- 2 tablespoons of glycerin
- 4 egg yolks
- A dash of sea salt
- ¼ teaspoon Xanthan gum
- 1 teaspoon scraped vanilla bean
- 2 cups heavy cream
- ½ cup Erythritol
- 1 ½ cups almond milk
- 3 ounces dark chocolate
- Liquid Stevia to taste

Directions:

1. Mix Stevia, almond milk, and heavy cream in a saucepan over low heat
2. Whisk and combine in a pan. In a mixing bowl beat egg yolks until they are smooth.
3. Check the temperature of the mix using a candy thermometer.
4. When the mix reaches 170^0 Fahrenheit remove it from the heat.
5. Pour the mix over the egg yolks. Mix well. Return to saucepan and heat over low heat.
6. Prepare an ice bath when the temperature reaches 175^0 Fahrenheit, remove from heat and mix with chocolate until smooth.
7. Place it over an ice bath and allow it to sit for 15 minutes then add in the remaining ingredients.
8. Add mix to ice cream maker and churn according to directions. Place in the freezer for 3 hours.

40) Mocha Coconut Ice Cream

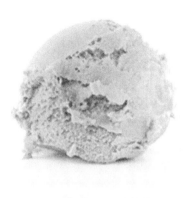

Servings: 8
Total Prep time: 4 hours

Ingredients:
- 4 cups of coconut milk
- 1 cup coconut cream
- 4 tablespoons of instant coffee
- 1 teaspoon of Xanthan gum
- 8 tablespoons of dark cocoa powder
- 8 tablespoons of Erythritol
- Liquid Stevia to taste

Directions:
1. Blend all the ingredients except for the gum.
2. Blend until smooth.
3. Eventually add in the Xanthan gum, blending mix until it becomes homogenous.
4. Pour your mix into your ice cream maker and churn according to directions.

41)   Coconut Cocoa Popsicles

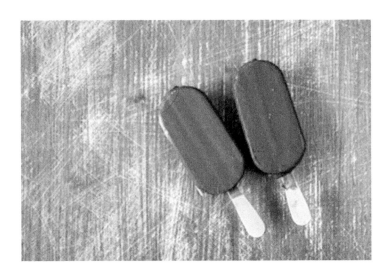

Servings: 8
Total Prep time: 2 hours

Ingredients:
- ¼ cup coconut, shredded
- 2 teaspoons vanilla extract
- 13 ounces coconut milk
- 2/3 cup cocoa powder
- Liquid Stevia to taste

Directions:
1. Blend your coconut milk, vanilla extract, cocoa powder, and sweetener until you have formed a smoothie.
2. Pour it into Popsicle molds and freeze until set.
3. Roll in coconut and enjoy!

42)   Swirly Peanut Butter Ice Cream

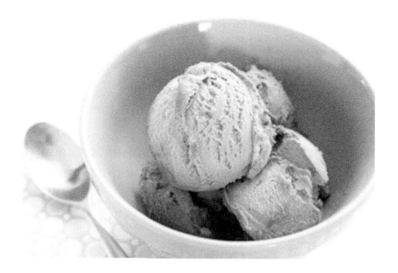

Servings: 8
Total Prep time: 4 hours

Ingredients:
- 2 ½ tablespoons of cocoa powder
- 1 ½ teaspoon of vanilla extract
- ¼ teaspoon sea salt
- 2/3 cups full-cream milk
- 6 tablespoons of butter
- 2 ½ tablespoons of avocado oil
- 4 eggs Stevia to taste

For Swirl:
- 5 tablespoons of coconut oil
- Stevia to taste
- 2/3 cup peanut butter, smooth

Directions:
1. Separate egg yolks, from the two eggs

2. You will need two egg yolks and two whole eggs for this recipe.
3. Add all the ingredients into your blender.
4. Blend until smooth.
5. Add to your ice cream maker and churn according to directions.
6. Whisk together your ingredients for the swirl and place in your fridge.
7. Before you turn off the ice cream maker, add in your swirl and allow it to roll for an additional minute.

43)   Cinnamon Roll Chocolate Ice Cream

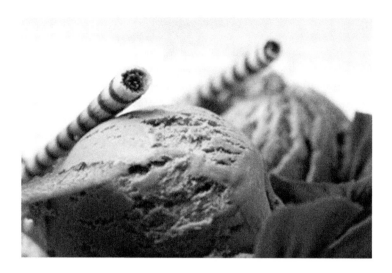

Servings: 8
Total Prep time: 4 hours

Ingredients:

- 2 tablespoons of cinnamon, ground
- 4 teaspoons of vanilla extract
- 27 ounces of coconut milk
- ½ cup dark chocolate, grated
- 2 teaspoons of additional cinnamon, ground
- Erythritol to taste

Directions:

1. Blend all your ingredients apart from the 2 teaspoons of additional cinnamon.
2. Pour mix into your ice cream maker and churn until the combination is set.
3. Freeze the mix and then scoop and serve with sprinkling top with remaining cinnamon.

44)   Chocolate Chip Ice Cream with Vanilla Bean

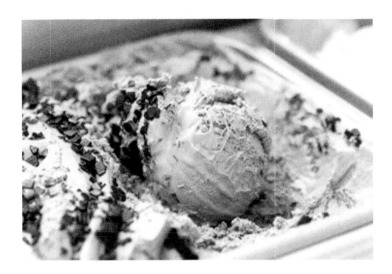

Servings: 8
Total Prep time: 3 hours

Ingredients:
- 1 cup half and half
- 1 cup unsweetened chocolate chips
- A dash of sea salt
- 3 egg yolks
- 1 teaspoon glycerin
- 1 tablespoon of scraped vanilla bean
- Stevia or Erythritol to taste

Directions:
1. Blend all your ingredients, except for the chocolate chips, blend them until smooth.
2. Add them to your ice cream maker and churn until set.
3. Before you turn off your ice cream maker, add in the chocolate chips and allow it to run for an additional two minutes.

45) Peanut Butter Cup on a Stick

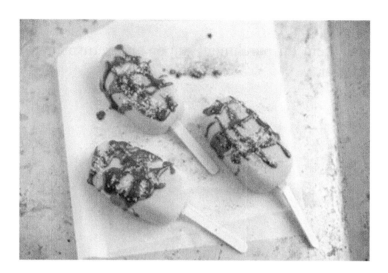

Servings: 8
Total Prep time: 3 hours

Ingredients:
- ½ teaspoon vanilla extract
- 1/3 cup peanut butter, smooth 2/3 cup heavy cream
- 1/3 cup full cream milk
- Sweetener to taste

Coating:
- 1/3 cup (Medium chain triglycerides) oil
- 2/3 cup dark chocolate, grated
- Sweetener to taste

Directions:
1. Whip your cream until it is light and frothy. Your cream is done when stiff peaks form.
2. Gently fold the rest of your ingredients into it.
3. Pour into molds and freeze until set.
4. Melt the oil and chocolate together over a double boiler.

5. Mix in your sweetener and remove from heat.
6. Remove popsicles from the freezer and dip into the chocolate mix.
7. Set them on parchment paper and return them to the freezer.
8. Enjoy

46)   Matcha Ice Cream

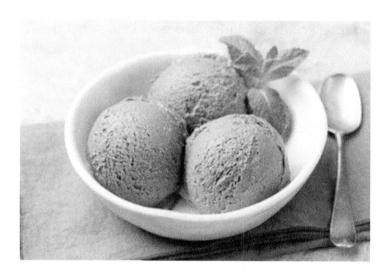

Servings: 8
Total Prep time: 3 hours

Ingredients:
- 3 tablespoons of coconut oil
- 2 tablespoons of Matcha green tea powder
- 27 ounces of coconut milk
- ¼ teaspoon of Guar gum
- Stevia to taste

Directions:
1. Pour the coconut milk into a saucepan and set on low heat.
2. Add in the Matcha green tea powder and begin to stir. Do not allow the mix to boil.
3. Once it has completely dissolved the milk will turn green in color.
4. Pour mixture into mixing bowl and set over an ice bath.
5. Add in the rest of the ingredients and stir.

6. Cool mix at room temperature, pour it into the ice cream maker and churn until set.
7. Freeze, scoop and enjoy this cool keto sweet treat!

47) Banana Chocolate Chip Ice Cream

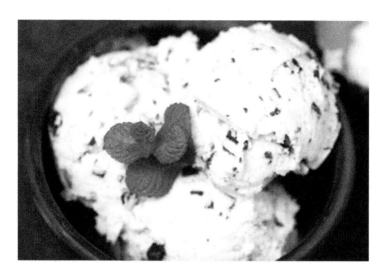

Servings: 8
Total Prep time: 4hours

Ingredients:

- 3 ounces of chocolate chips, dark, unsweetened
- 4 bananas
- 1 cup full cream milk
- 3 egg yolks
- 2 tablespoons of glycerin
- ½ teaspoon of Xanthan gum
- ½ teaspoon vanilla extract
- 1 cup heavy whipping cream
- 5 tablespoons of butter
- Stevia to taste

Directions:

1. Freeze the bananas overnight. The next day slice your bananas into rounds.
2. Place them into your food processor and blend until smooth and frothy.
3. Set your banana mix aside.
4. In a saucepan add in the butter, and Stevia cook over low heat, bring to a boil.
5. Remove it from heat and stir in the vanilla extract.
6. Return to heat and add in the heavy whipping cream, stirring constantly.
7. When it has reached 170^0 Fahrenheit stir in the milk and continue to stir it.
8. In a mixing bowl whisk the egg yolks until they are smooth.
9. Pour your milk mix over your eggs and whisk. Return to saucepan and heat.
10. Remove from heat and add in the banana mix, stir until it thickens.
11. Add mix to your ice cream maker and churn until it sets. Just before you turn off ice cream maker, add in chocolate chips and churn for another additional minute.
12. Freeze, and enjoy!

48)   Spicy Pumpkin Latte Ice Cream

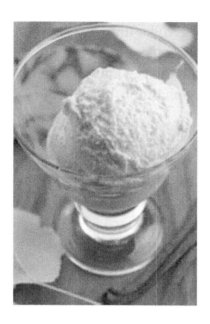

Servings: 8
Total Prep time: 4 hours

Ingredients:
- ½ cup pumpkin seeds
- 4 cups full cream milk
- 2 teaspoons of Maple extract
- 6 egg yolks
- 4 tablespoons of salted butter
- 1 teaspoon Xanthan gum
- 1 cup pumpkin puree
- 1 cup cottage cheese
- Stevia to taste

Directions:
1. Place your saucepan over medium heat and melt the butter.

2. Add in the pumpkin seeds and cook until they are toasted. Remove them from heat and set aside.
3. Beat your egg yolks until they are creamy and smooth, add in your sweetener.
4. Pour milk into the egg and mix well.
5. Add in the remaining ingredients except for pumpkin seeds.
6. Mix using an immersion blender.
7. Pour into your ice cream maker and churn until it is set.
8. Just before you shut off the ice cream maker, add in the pumpkin seeds and churn for an additional 5 minutes.
9. Freeze, and enjoy!

49)   Almond Rose Ice Cream

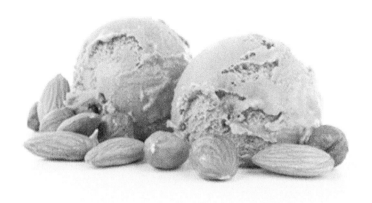

Servings: 8
Total Prep time: 7 hours

Ingredients:
- ½ cup raw almonds
- 4 tablespoons of rose water
- 2 cups heavy whipping cream
- 1 cup almond milk
- Erythritol to taste

Directions:
1. Soak the almonds in water overnight. Peel them and drain the water and pat them dry with some paper towel.
2. Pulse them to a powder using your food processor.
3. Beat the cream until it is stiff and forms peaks.
4. Add milk to it and beat it again.
5. Fold in the remaining ingredients.
6. Place in a metallic container and place in the freezer.

7. After about two hours the ice cream should be solidified.
8. Stir it thoroughly and return it to the freezer.
9. After another two hours stir it again and return to the freezer, do this process three times.

50)   Minty Avocado Ice Cream

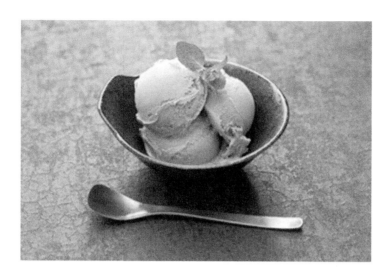

Servings: 8
Total Prep time: 12 hours

Ingredients:

- 4 bananas
- 2 avocados
- 2/3 cup cocoa nibs
- ½ teaspoon Xanthan gum
- ¼ teaspoon peppermint extract
- Stevia to taste

Directions:

1. Freeze the bananas overnight. The next day slice them into rounds.
2. Peel and dice your avocados.
3. Place both the avocados and bananas in your food processor.
4. Blend on low.

5. Due to the bananas being frozen, the mixture will develop a mousse-like consistency.
6. Keep blending until it becomes light and frothy.
7. Stir in the remaining ingredients and transfer it into the freezer and freeze overnight.

POPSICLES

51)   Cheesecake Frozen Yogurt Pops

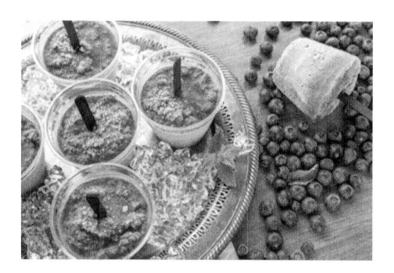

Servings: 6
Total Prep time: 4 hours 25 minutes

Ingredients:
- 1 Packet Graham Crackers
- 8oz Can Condensed Milk
- 18oz Blueberries
- 1 Cup Greek Yogurt

Directions
1. Put the graham crackers in a food processor and pulse.
2. Add 2 tablespoons of the condensed milk and blitz again until the crumbs come together and begin to form a ball
3. Divide between 8 paper cups and press down firmly so that the crumbs hold their shape.   Place half the

blueberries, condensed milk, and yogurt in a blender and blend until smooth and silky in consistency

4. Add the remaining blueberries and pulse briefly to chop roughly
5. Pour into the paper cups on top of the breadcrumbs
6. Place a layer of cling film over each cup and then insert a wooden Popsicle stick in each one. The cling film will help to hold the stick in place
7. Freeze for 4 hours and then serve

52)   Berry Melon Pops

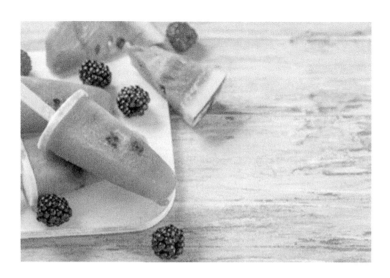

Servings: 5
Total Prep time: 4 hours 15 minutes

Ingredients

- 3 cups seedless watermelon, cubed
- 1 cup fresh blackberries
- 1 cup sparkling water
- 1 tablespoon fresh mint

Directions

1. Place all ingredients in a blender. Blend until pureed and smooth.
2. Transfer the puree to ice pop molds and place in the freezer.
3. Freeze for at least 4 hours or overnight for best results.

53) Frozen Vanilla Banana Pops.

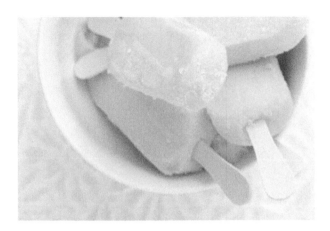

Servings: 4
Total Prep time: 4 hours 10 minutes

Ingredients
- 2 medium bananas
- ½ cup unsweetened coconut milk
- ½ teaspoon cinnamon
- 1 teaspoon honey (optional)
- ½ cup sugar-free vanilla Greek yogurt
- 1 teaspoon vanilla extract

Directions
1. In a blender, combine the bananas, coconut milk, cinnamon, and honey.
2. Blend until smooth and transfer the mixture to a bowl.
3. Mix the yogurt and vanilla extract before adding the yogurt to the banana mixture.
4. Spoon the mixture into ice pop molds and place in the freezer.
5. Freeze for at least 4 hours, or overnight for best results.

54) Mango Gelatin pops

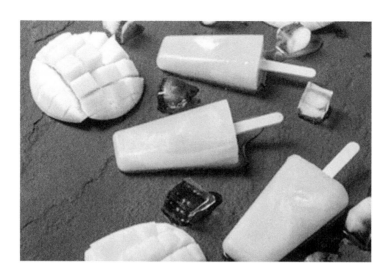

Servings: 5
Total Prep time: 4 hours 10 minutes

Ingredients

- 1 3 oz box sugar-free orange flavored gelatin
- 1 cup boiling water
- 1 cup cold sparkling water
- 1 cup fresh mango, cubed
- 2 teaspoons fresh grated ginger

Directions

1. In a bowl combine the orange gelatin and boiling water. Stir to dissolve.
2. Add the cold sparkling water and set aside to cool.
3. In a blender combine the mango and grated ginger.
4. Blend to desired consistency, either pureeing for a smooth ice pop.
5. Add the gelatin mixture to the blender and pulse quickly once or twice to blend.

6. Transfer to ice pop molds and place in the freezer.
7. Freeze for at least 4 hours, or overnight for best results.

55) Choco Fudge Pops

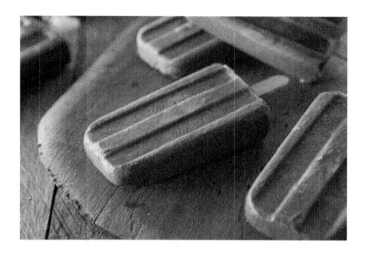

Servings: 4
Total Prep time: 12 hours

Ingredients
- 1 cup sugar-free vanilla Greek yogurt
- 1 cup unsweetened almond milk
- 1 tablespoon dark cocoa powder
- 1 teaspoon vanilla extract
- 2 teaspoons cinnamon
- 2 tablespoons extra dark or sugar-free chocolate chips (optional)

Directions
1. In a blender combine the vanilla Greek yogurt, almond milk, cocoa powder, vanilla extract, and cinnamon. Blend until creamy.
2. Spoon a few chocolate chips (optional) into each of the ice pop molds before topping with the chocolate mixture.
3. Place in the freezer and freeze overnight for best results.

56)   Strawberries and Cream Bars

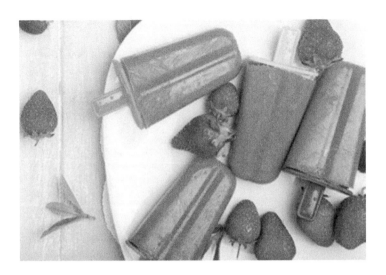

Servings: 4
Total Prep time: 12 hours

Ingredients

- 2 cups fresh strawberries, quartered
- 1 cup sugar-free vanilla yogurt
- ½ cup unsweetened coconut milk
- 1 teaspoon vanilla extract

Directions

1. Combine the strawberries, vanilla yogurt, coconut milk and vanilla extract in a blender. Blend until desired consistency is reached, leaving a few chunks of strawberries, if desired.
2. Pour the mixture into ice pop molds and freeze overnight for best results.

57)   Fruit Salad Pops

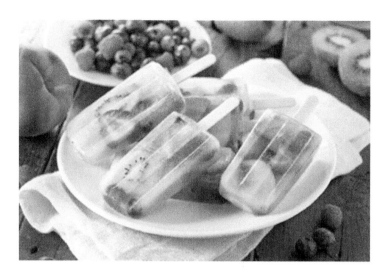

Servings: 5
Total Prep time: 12 hours

Ingredients
- ½ cup mango, cubed
- 1 kiwi fruit, peeled and sliced
- ½ cup fresh raspberries
- ½ cup fresh peaches, peeled and cubed
- 1 cup naturally flavored lemon sparkling water
- 1 tablespoon lime juice
- 1 teaspoon lime zest

Directions
1. Carefully arrange the prepared fruit into the ice pops molds.
2. Pack more fruit into the mold for a chunkier texture.
3. Combine the sparkling lemon water, lime juice, and lime zest.

4. Add the sparkling water mixture to each mold, tapping gently to make sure the liquid surrounds the fruit.
5. Place in the freezer and freeze overnight for best results.

58)   Pistachio Pops

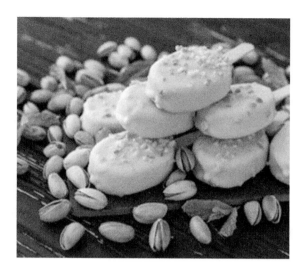

Servings: 4
Total Prep time: 4 hours 1 minute

Ingredients

- ½ cup sugar-free vanilla Greek yogurt
- ½ cup heavy cream
- 2 tablespoons sugar-free pistachio pudding mix
- ½ teaspoon orange extract
- ½ teaspoon cardamom
- ¼ cup crushed pistachios

Directions

1. In a blender, combine the yogurt, heavy cream, pudding mix, orange extract, and cardamom.
2. Blend until smooth and creamy.
3. Pour the mixture into the ice pop molds.
4. Sprinkle a generous portion of crushed pistachios into each mold before placing in the freezer.
5. Freeze for at least 4 hours, or overnight for best results.

SORBETS

59)   Blueberry Sorbet

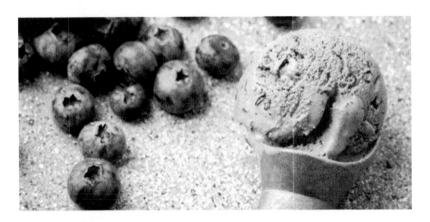

Servings: 5
Total Prep time: 6 hours 10 minutes

Ingredients:
- 180g blueberries
- 90ml coconut milk
- 1 egg
- ½ banana
- 2 tablespoons honey

Directions:
1. Wash blueberries and dry them with a paper towel, transfer to a mixing bowl.
2. Mash banana with a fork and add to blueberries.
3. Pour coconut milk, add honey and blend everything with an electrical blender.
4. Separate egg white from the yolk and beat egg white to stiff peaks.
5. Add the beaten egg to the mixture, pour it into the container and freeze for at least 6 hours.

60) Pomegranate Sorbet

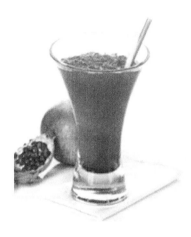

Servings: 4
Total Prep time: 5 hours 15 minutes

Ingredients:
- 180ml pomegranate juice
- 160g blueberries
- 120ml water
- 60g sugar
- 2 tablespoons cornstarch
- Pinch salt

Directions:
1. Pre-heat a saucepan over high heat, pour pomegranate juice.
2. Bring to a boil and turn to low heat. Cook until the juice reduces by ¼.
3. Add blueberries and cook for 5 more minutes.
4. Puree the mixture with an electric blender.

5. Pre-heat another saucepan with 80ml water over medium heat, add sugar.
6. Bring to a boil and swirl by the handle to let the sugar dissolve. Do not stir.
7. Turn to high heat and cook until the mixture thickens. Turn to low heat.
8. Combine the remaining water with cornstarch and salt, whisk well until cornstarch dissolves and add to syrup.
9. Cook for 1 more minute and fruit puree and mix thoroughly.
10. Chill the mixture in the ice water for 10 minutes, blend it.
11. Transfer to a container and put in the freezer for 5 hours.

61)   Peach Sorbet

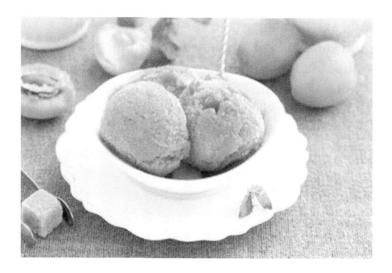

Servings: 4
Total Prep time: 5 hours 15 minutes

Ingredients:
- 3 peaches
- 380ml water
- 60g sugar
- 50g raspberries
- ½ lemon
- 2 teaspoons gelatin
- Pinch salt

Directions:
1. Combine gelatin with 130ml water to make it soft.
2. Peel off the peaches, remove the cores and cut into cubes.
3. Combine cubed peaches with raspberries and puree them with an electrical blender.

4. Pre-heat a saucepan with the remaining water, add the puree.
5. Add salt and sugar and stir until it dissolves.
6. Add softened gelatin and cook for one more minute.
7. Squeeze 1 tablespoon lemon juice to the saucepan, stir.
8. Chill the mixture in the ice water for 5-10 minutes, stir it thoroughly and transfer to a container.
9. Freeze for 5 hours.

62)   Raspberry sorbet

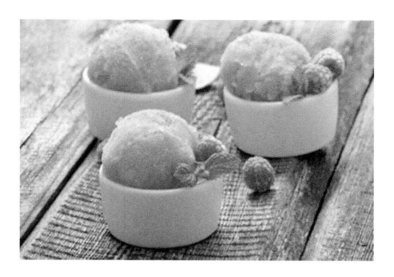

Servings: 5
Total Prep time: 6 hours 10 minutes

Ingredients:

- 150g raspberries
- 1 egg
- 80ml coconut milk
- ½ banana
- ½ lemon
- 1 tablespoon honey

Directions:

1. Pour coconut milk into the bowl, add raspberries and honey.
2. Squeeze lemon and add 1 tablespoon juice to coconut milk.
3. Cut banana into pieces, transfer to the bowl and blend with an electrical blender until you get a homogenous structure.

4. Separate egg white from the yolk, whisk egg white to stiff peaks.
5. Add blended mixture to whisked eggs, mix well.
6. Transfer the mixture to the container and freeze for at least 6 hours.

63)   Strawberry sorbet

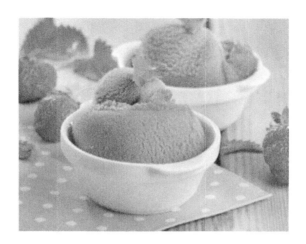

Servings: 8
Total Prep time: 1 hour 20 minutes

Ingredients:
- 500g strawberries
- 240g sugar
- 250ml water
- 1 lemon

Directions:
1. Bring water to a boil in a saucepan. Remove from heat.
2. Add sugar and mix well until it dissolves.
3. Squeeze juice from lemon and pour it to water, mix well.
4. Pour the syrup into the container and put it in the fridge for 1-2 hours.
5. Puree the strawberries with an electrical blender.
6. Add cooled syrup to the puree and blend with an electric blender.
7. Transfer the sorbet to the container and freeze for 1 more hour.

64)   Avocado sorbet

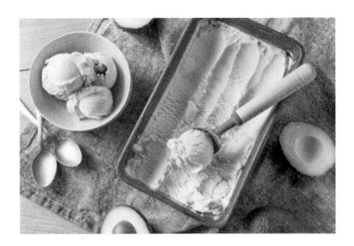

Servings: 4
Total Prep time: 11 hours

Ingredients:
- 200ml almond milk
- 100g Swerve sweetener
- 2 avocados
- 1 teaspoon mango extract

Directions:
1. Peel off avocados and remove cores. Mash it with a fork and put in the bowl.
2. Pour almond milk into the bowl, mix well.
3. Add sweetener and mango extract; combine all the ingredients with a mixer.
4. Chill the mixture in the ice water for 15 minutes.
5. Blend the chilled mixture with an electric blender for 20 minutes.
6. Transfer to a container and put it in the freezer for 10 hours.

65)   Easy banana sorbet

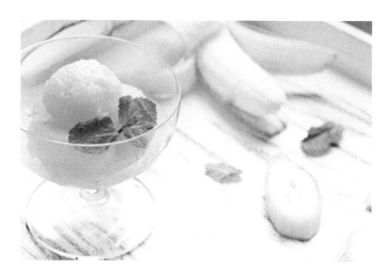

Servings: 4
Total Prep time: 6 hours 20 minutes

Ingredients:
- 2 bananas 250ml
- water 100g sugar

Directions:
1. Pre-heat a saucepan over medium heat, pour water.
2. Add sugar, bring to a boil and stir until the sugar dissolves to get syrup.
3. Chill the syrup in the ice water for 5 minutes.
4. Chop bananas and puree them with an electrical blender.
5. Combine banana puree and chilled syrup, mix thoroughly to get a homogenous structure.
6. Put the mixture in the freezer for 3 hours; blend it with an electric blender for 10 minutes.
7. Return to the freezer for 3 more hours.

66)   Melon sorbet

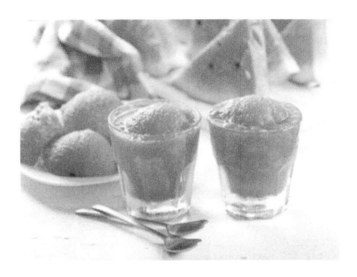

Servings: 4
Total Prep time: 2hours 10 minutes

Ingredients:
- 600g melon
- 230g sugar
- 170ml water
- Pinch of salt

Directions:
1. Pre-heat water over medium heat for about 3 minutes until the water starts steaming.
2. Add sugar and mix thoroughly until it dissolves.
   3) Cool the syrup in the fridge for at least 1 hour.
3. Peel off melon and cut into pieces, add cooled syrup and puree with an electric blender.
4. Add salt and mix well.
5. Transfer puree to a container and freeze for 1-2 hours.

67)   Strawberry cinnamon sorbet

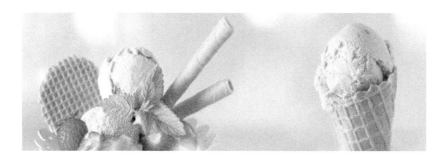

Servings: 4
Total Prep time: 3 hours 25 minutes

Ingredients:
- 750ml yogurt
- 130g sugar
- 50g strawberries
- 1 lemon
- 1 teaspoon vanilla extract
- 1 teaspoon cinnamon
- Pinch salt

Directions:
1. Combine yogurt with sugar, vanilla extract, salt, and cinnamon, whisk thoroughly with a hand whisk.
2. Zest lemon and squeeze juice. Add lemon juice and 1 teaspoon lemon zest to a mixture. Chill the mixture in the freezer for 10 minutes.
3. Wash strawberries and dry them with paper towels, chop finely.
4. Blend the chilled mixture with an electric blender for 10 minutes, add chopped strawberries and blend for 2 more minutes.
5. Transfer the mixture to a container and freeze for 2-4 hours.

68)   Grapefruit sorbet

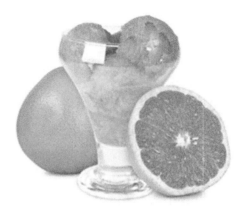

Servings: 4
Total Prep time: 5 hours 10 minutes

Ingredients:
- 250ml water
- 100g sugar
- 2 grapefruit
- 2 teaspoons tarragon
- Pinch of salt

Directions:
1. Pre-heat a saucepan over medium heat, pour water.
2. Add sugar, tarragon and salt and heat for 5 minutes frequently stirring until sugar dissolves.
3. Remove the mixture from heat and let it steep for 1 hour.
4. Squeeze juice from grapefruit; add it to the mixture when it steeped.
5. Whisk the mixture with a mixer; chill it in the fridge for 3 hours.
6. Blend it with an electrical mixture when chilled, transfer to a container.
7. Put the mixture in the freezer for 4 hours.

69) Coconut ginger sorbet

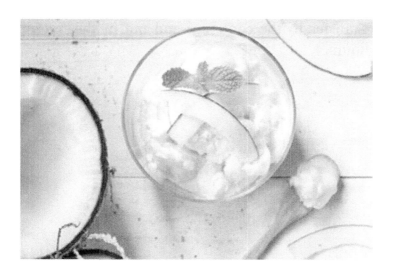

Servings: 5
Total Prep time: 5 hours 10 minutes

Ingredients:

- 420ml coconut milk
- 180ml water
- 80g sugar
- 30g coconut flakes
- 1 teaspoon ginger
- ¼ teaspoon vanilla
- Pinch salt

Directions:

1. Pre-heat a saucepan over medium heat, pour water.
2. Add sugar, ginger, and salt to water, mix well.
3. Cook for 3-5 minutes, stirring occasionally. Remove from heat and cool for 1 hour. Pour coconut milk in the bowl; add coconut flakes and vanilla combine well.

4. Using a sieve, add cooled mixture to the coconut milk. Whisk thoroughly.
5. Transfer to the container and put in the freezer for 5 hours.

70)   Mint avocado sorbet

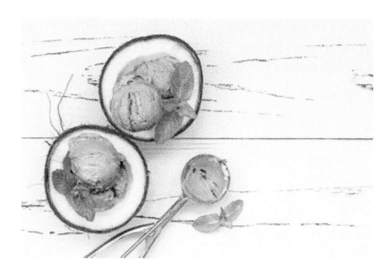

Servings: 5
Total Prep time: 6 hours 10 minutes

Ingredients:

- 80ml coconut milk
- 3 avocados
- 2 eggs
- ¼ melon
- ½ lemon Bunch mint
- 2 tablespoons honey

Directions:

1. Remove the skin and stone from avocados, cut into pieces and place in a bowl. Remove the skin from melon, dice and add to avocados.
2. Squeeze lemon and transfer to the bowl with mint and honey.
3. Pour coconut milk into the bowl and blend with an electric blender for 2-3 minutes.

ICE CREAM RECIPE BOOK

4. Separate egg whites from yolks beat egg whites to stiff peaks and combine with the blended mixture.
5. Transfer the mixture to the container and put it into the freezer for 6 hours.
6. Cut into slices before serving.

71)Rhubarb orange sorbet

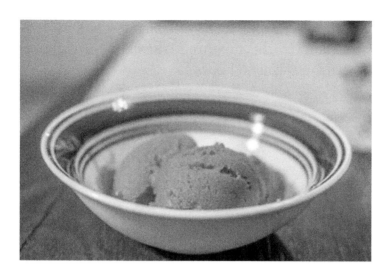

Servings: 5
Total Prep time: 6 hours 10 minutes

Ingredients:
- 4 oranges
- 5 rhubarb stalks
- 1 egg
- 1 tablespoon honey
- ½ teaspoon vanilla extract

Directions:
1. Pre-heat a pan over medium heat.
2. Remove the leaves of rhubarb stalks, trim ends and cut into pieces. Transfer to the pan. Squeeze oranges to get about 250ml juice. Pour the squeezed juice to the chopped rhubarb. Add honey and vanilla, mix well, cover with the lid and cook for 4-6 minutes. Remove from heat and cool to the room temperature.

3. Blend the cooled mixture with an electrical blender until you get a homogenous structure.
4. Separate egg white from yolk beat egg yolk to stiff peaks and scold in the mixture. Transfer to a container and freeze for at least 6 hours.

72) Pinacolada sorbet

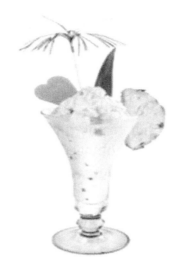

Servings: 4
Total Prep time: 4 hours 30 minutes

Ingredients:
- 1 pineapple
- ½ lemon
- 250ml coconut milk
- 60ml water
- 100g sugar
- 30g coconut flakes
- 1 teaspoon ginger
- ¼ teaspoon vanilla extract
- Pinch salt

Directions:
1. Heat water on a saucepan over medium heat
2. Add sugar and salt, heat for 5 minutes, occasionally stirring until the sugar dissolves. Chill the syrup in the ice water for 5-10 minutes stirring from time to time.

3. Peel the pineapple, remove the core and cut it into cubes.
4. Squeeze juice from a lemon, zest it.
5. Add 3 tablespoons lemon juice to the cubed pineapple.
6. Puree the pineapple with an electrical blender. Strain through a sieve.
7. Add syrup, coconut milk, coconut flakes, 1 teaspoon lemon zest and salt to the puree. Mix with an electric mixer until you get a homogenous structure.
8. Freeze for at least 6 hours, blend again and freeze for 4 more hours.

73)   Basil and lime ice

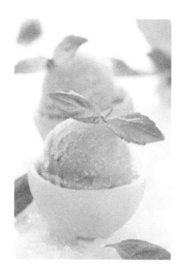

Servings: 3
Total Prep time: 3 hours 10 minutes

Ingredients:
- Bunch basil leaves
- 120ml coconut milk
- 120ml water
- 5 limes
- 2 tablespoons honey

Directions:
1. Wash basil leaves, dry them with paper towels and chop.
2. Squeeze limes to get 120ml juice, pour juice to chopped basil.
3. Add water, coconut milk, and honey; blend with an electric blender to get a homogenous structure.
4. Transfer the mixture to the container and freeze for 2 hours.

5. Break the chilled mixture into pieces with a fork and freeze for 40 more minutes. Repeat it if necessary until you have crushed ice.

FROZEN YOGURTS, GELATOS & GRANITAS

74) Avocado Frozen Yogurt

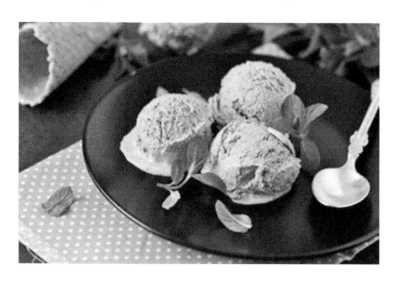

Servings: 4
Total Prep time: 40 minutes

Ingredients:

- 1 large, ripe avocado (peeled, pitted)
- 2 cups plain yogurt
- ½ cup whole milk
- ½ tsp pure vanilla extract
- 4 tbsp. sugar

Directions:

1. Place the avocado flesh along with the yogurt, milk, vanilla extract to a blender and process until silky smooth.
2. Add the sweetening a little at a time, until you achieved your desired level of sweetness. Process briefly to combine

3. Transfer the mixture to your ice cream maker and churn to manufacturer's instructions. Enjoy right away as soft serve, or place in the freezer for 30 minutes, this will give you a firmer consistency.

75)   Blackberry frozen yogurt

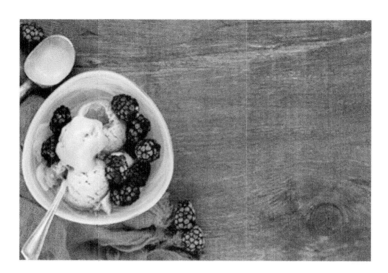

Servings: 4
Total Prep time: 1 hour 15minutes

Ingredients:
- 2 cups fresh washed and dried blackberries
- ½ cup honey
- 7 whole mint leaves
- 3 cups plain Greek yogurt
- 3 tbsp. mint leaves (finely chopped)

Directions:
1. Add the blackberries along with the honey to a food blender and on high speed, process until pureed.
2. Add the mint and process till the mint leaves are no longer visible.
3. Pour the mixture through a mesh strainer to strain the seeds and any stray pieces of mint leaves.
4. As soon as the fruit mixture is strained, add the yogurt to the mixing bowl and using a whisk, combine.

5. Add the chopped mint leaves to the yogurt mixture, stir in, using a whisk.

6. As soon as the chopped mint is evenly incorporated, transfer to an ice cream machine and process according to the manufacturer's instructions.

7. Transfer to a freezer-safe container and freeze for an hour before serving.

76) Blueberry Frozen Yogurt

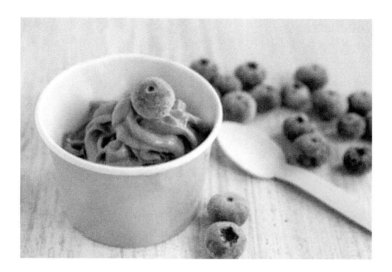

Servings: 6
Total Prep time: 1 hour 10 minutes

Ingredients

- 2 cups plain low-fat yogurt
- 2 cups fresh blueberries
- 1 firm banana, cut
- 2 tbsp. sugar or honey
- 1 tsp. lime juice
- 1/2 tsp. lime zest

Directions

1. Blend all ingredients in a food processor; make sure that the sugar is dissolved.
2. Use an ice cream maker according to instructions to make frozen yogurt, or pour the mixture into a covered container and let freeze for an hour before eating.

3. Before serving to keep the frozen yogurt at cold room temperature for it not to be too hard. Garnish with fresh blueberries.

77)   Apple Frozen Yogurt

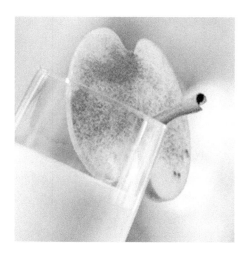

Servings: 6
Total Prep time: 1 hour 10 minutes

Ingredients

- 2 cups plain Greek yogurt
- 1/2 cup heavy cream
- 1 large firm sour apple, peeled and cut
- 1/2 cup honey
- 2 tsp ground cinnamon

Directions

1. In a food processor, puree apple until smooth, blend in yogurt, honey, and cinnamon.
2. Use an ice cream maker according to instructions to make frozen yogurt, or pour the mixture into a covered container and let freeze for an hour before eating.
3. Garnish with apple slices, cinnamon, and honey.
4. Enjoy.

78) Chocolate Frozen Yogurt with Peanut Butter

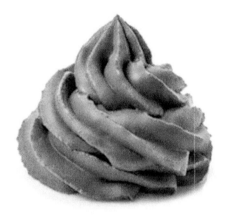

Servings: 3
Total Prep time: 1 hour 10 minutes

Ingredients

- 2 cups plain or vanilla low-fat yogurt
- 1/2 cup semi-sweet chocolate chips
- 3 tbsp. white chocolate chips
- 1/3 cup creamy peanut butter
- 1/3 cup brown sugar
- 1/3 heavy cream

Directions

1. In a saucepan, combine the sugar, cream and chocolate chips.
2. Stir over low heat until sugar and chocolate chips melted.
3. Let the chocolate sauce cool a bit, and then add peanut butter and yogurt.
4. After the mixture is entirely relaxed - add white chocolate chips and mix thoroughly. Use an ice cream

maker according to instructions to make frozen yogurt, or pour the mixture into a covered container and let freeze for an hour before eating.

5. Defrost slightly before serving.
6. Garnish with melted chocolate or whipped cream. Frozen

79) Vanilla Cherry Ice Cream

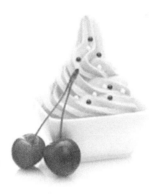

Servings: 5
Total Prep time: 1 hour

Ingredients:
- 2 cups heavy cream
- 1 cup milk
- 3/4 cup white sugar
- 1 tbsp. vanilla extract
- 1 tsp. almond extract
- 2 cups fresh cherries, pits removed and cut in half

Directions:
1. Combine the cream, milk, and sugar in a bowl.
2. Stir until the sugar is completely dissolved.
3. Stir in the vanilla and almond extract. Add the cherries.
4. Pour the mixture into an ice cream maker and churn according to the manufacturer's instructions.
5. Transfer to a freezer-safe container and freeze for at least 2 hours before serving.

80)   Instant Berry Frozen Yogurt

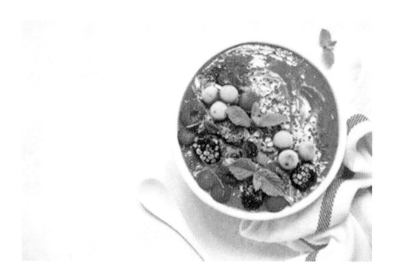

Servings: 4
Total Prep time: 15 minutes

Ingredients:
- 8oz Frozen Mixed Berries
- 8oz Greek Yogurt
- 1 Tbsp Honey

Directions
1. Place the frozen berries, yogurt and honey in a blender and blend for 30 seconds.
2. The mixture should be in a ball form and have the consistency of ice cream.
3. Serve immediately

81)   Classic Vanilla Frozen Yogurt

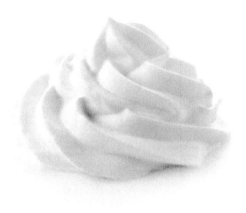

Servings: 8
Total Prep time: 1 hour 5 minutes

Ingredients
- 2 cups plain low-fat yogurt
- 1/2 cup sugar
- 1/2 tsp. vanilla

Directions
1. Mix or blend all ingredients. Make the sugar dissolve. Taste and add in as much sugar as seems reasonable to you.
2. Use an ice cream maker according to instructions to make vanilla yogurt, or pour the mixture into a covered container and let freeze for an hour before eating.
3. Before serving keep the frozen yogurt at cold room temperature for not being too hard.

82)   Shortcake Frozen Yogurt

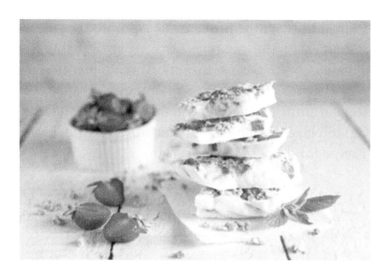

Servings: 8
Total Prep time: 4 hours 20 minutes

Ingredients:
- 1 Punnet Strawberries, hulled
- 2 Cups Greek Yogurt
- 1 Can Condensed Milk
- 1 Tsp Vanilla Bean Paste
- 1 Cup Double Cream
- 8 Pieces Shortbread, crushed with a rolling pin

Directions
1. Make a puree with the strawberries by placing them in a blender and blending to a smooth paste. (Remember to keep a handful of strawberries aside for garnish)
2. Add the Greek yogurt, the condensed milk and the vanilla paste to the blender and pulse to combine thoroughly

3. Whip the cream in a bowl until soft peaks form. Add 1/3 of the strawberry puree and mix.
4. Repeat until all the puree is incorporated.
5. Pour 1/4 of the mixture into a plastic container then sprinkle over 1/4 of the shortbread pieces and extra strawberries. Then cover with another layer of mixture.
6. Repeat until all the ingredients are used up. Make sure the top layer is made up of biscuits and strawberries.
7. Freeze for 4 hours before serving

83) Vanilla Gelato

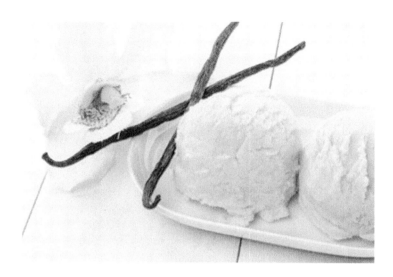

Servings: 7
Total Prep time: 1 hour

Ingredients:
- 5 egg yolks
- 1/2 cup sugar
- 2 cups milk
- 1 cup heavy cream
- seeds from 1 vanilla pod

Directions:
1. In a bowl, mix the egg yolks with the sugar and vanilla seeds until creamy and pale then stir in the milk and place the bowl over a water bath.
2. Cook the custard until thick and it coats the back of a spoon.
3. Remove from heat and let it cool to room temperature before proceeding to next step. Once chilled, stir in the heavy cream, whipped to soft peaks stage.

4. Spoon the mixture into your ice cream maker and freeze according to manufacturer's instructions.

5. Enjoy.

84) Chocolate Gelato

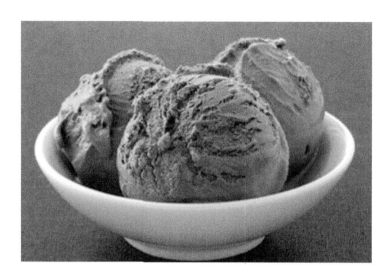

Servings: 10
Total Prep time: 1 hour

Ingredients:

- 5 egg yolks
- 2 cups milk
- 2 tablespoons cocoa powder
- 3oz dark chocolate
- 2/3 cup sugar
- 1/2 teaspoon vanilla extract
- 1 pinch of salt

Directions:

1. In a small saucepan, mix the egg yolks with the cocoa powder, sugar, and milk and simmer on low heat until thick and it coats the back of a spoon.
2. Remove from heat and while it's still hot, stir in the chocolate and mix until melted. Add the vanilla and let the custard cool.

3. Whip the heavy cream to soft peaks and fold it into the custard.
4. Transfer the mixture into your ice cream maker and churn according to your machine's instructions.
5. Enjoy.

85)   Espresso Granita

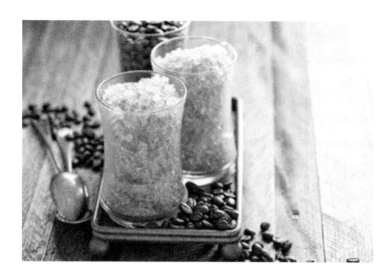

Servings: 4
Total Prep time: 1 hour

Ingredients
- 2 cups strongly brewed espresso
- 1 teaspoon vanilla extract
- 1 12 ounces can unsweetened full-fat coconut milk
- 1 tablespoon shredded, unsweetened coconut

Directions
1. Brew and cool the espresso.
2. Place the unopened can of coconut milk in the refrigerator and chill for 2-4 hours.
3. Add the espresso and vanilla to a shallow baking pan and stir well.
4. Place the pan in the freezer. After one hour, remove the pan and stir or scrape with a fork.

5. Return the pan to the freezer and repeat once an hour until icy, slushy consistency forms.

6. When the granita is close to being done, remove the coconut milk from the refrigerator. Spoon out the thick coconut cream that has risen to the top, and place in a mixing bowl. Briefly beat on high speed to create a thick, fluffy coconut cream.

7. Serve the granita in well-chilled classes, topped with coconut cream and shredded coconut.

86) Lemon Gelato

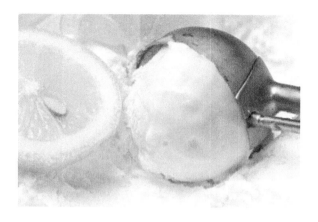

Servings: 4
Total Prep time: 1 hour

Ingredients:
- 1 cup heavy cream
- 1 1/2 cup milk
- zest and juice from 2 lemons
- 3/4 cup sugar
- 6 egg yolks

Directions:
1. In a heat-proof bowl, mix the yolks with the sugar until creamy and fluffy then stir in the milk.
2. Place the bowl over a double boiler and cook until heated through and it starts to thicken.
3. Remove from heat and stir in the lemon juice and lemon zest. Let it cool to room temperature then stir in the heavy cream, whipped to soft peaks stage.
4. Transfer the mixture into your ice cream maker and churn according to your machine's instructions.

87) Citrus Berry Granita

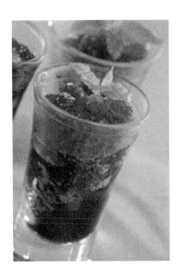

Servings: 4
Total Prep time: 3 hours

Ingredients
- 1 cup fresh strawberries, quartered
- 1 cup fresh raspberries
- ½ cup fresh blueberries
- ½ cup fresh orange juice (no additional sugar added)
- ½ cup fresh grapefruit juice (no extra sugar added)
- 1 tablespoon fresh lime juice

Directions
1. Add the strawberries, raspberries, and blueberries to a blender or food processor and blend until smooth.
2. Using a mesh strainer, press the berry puree to remove chunks and seeds

3. Place the berry puree into a shallow baking dish and stir in the orange juice, grapefruit juice, and lime juice. Mix well.
4. Shake or smooth out the puree so that the surface is even and place the pan in the freezer.
5. After an hour remove the pan from the freezer and stir or scrape with a fork. Continue doing this once an hour until mixture is icy and slushy.
6. Serve in well-chilled glasses.

88)   Mascarpone Gelato

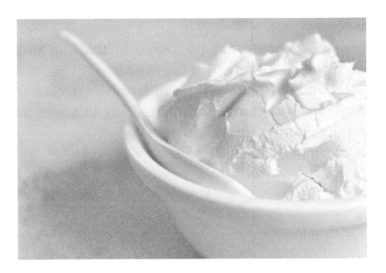

Servings: 8
Total Prep time: 10 minutes

Ingredients:
- 2 cups milk
- 2/3 cup sugar
- 2 tablespoons cornstarch
- 2 egg yolks
- 1 teaspoon vanilla extract
- 1 cup mascarpone cheese

Directions:
1. In a saucepan, mix the milk with the sugar, cornstarch and egg yolks and place on low heat.
2. Cook until it starts to thicken and it coats the back of a spoon then remove from heat and let it cool to room temperature.

3. When chilled, stir in the mascarpone cheese and vanilla then transfer into your ice cream maker and freeze according to your machine's instructions.

149

89)   Sour Apple Granita

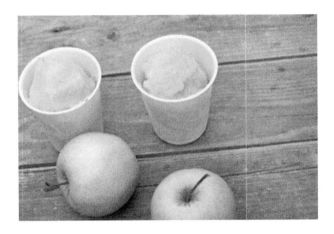

Servings: 4
Total Prep time: 4 hours 10 minutes

Ingredients
- 2 cups apples, peeled and chopped
- 1 cup fresh apple juice, no sugar added
- 2 tablespoons fresh lemon juice
- 1 teaspoon fresh ginger, grated

Directions
1. Place the apples and apple juice in a blender or food processor.
2. Blend until mixture is smooth and liquid.
3. Transfer the apple mixture to a shallow baking dish.
4. Add the lemon juice and fresh ginger. Mix well.
5. Place the pan in the freezer to chill.
6. Remove from the freezer after one hour. Stir with a fork and return to the fridge.
7. Repeat this once every hour until mixture is slushy and icy. Serve in well-chilled glasses.

VEGAN ICE CREAMS

90) Dairy-Free Ice Cream

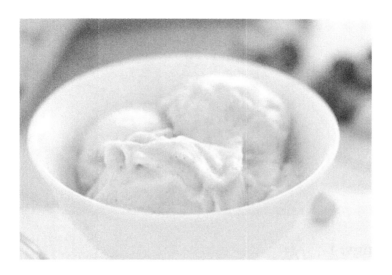

Servings: 8
Total Prep time: 4 hours 10 minutes

Ingredients:
- 1 cup soy milk
- 2 Tbsp sugar
- 1 tsp vanilla extract

Directions:
1. Mix all of the ingredients and add to the smaller bag.
2. Shake the mix and freeze for 4 hours.
3. Enjoy

91) Vegan Peanut Butter Ice

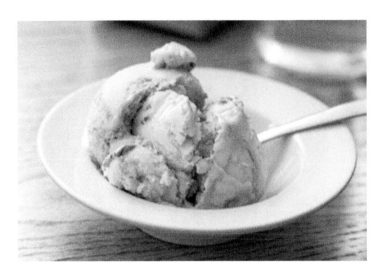

Servings: 1
Total Prep time: 20 minutes

Ingredients
- 2 1/2 teaspoons stevia
- 4 cups ice cubes
- 1/4 cup crunchy peanut butter
- 1 cup soy milk
- 2 teaspoons carob powder

Directions
1. Place the soymilk and peanut butter together in the jar of a blender.
2. Blend until just combined.
3. Add in the carob powder and stevia and blend for a few more minutes.
4. Add in the ice cubes and blend until it gets to slush like texture.
5. Serve immediately and enjoy.

92)   Cherry Ice Slush

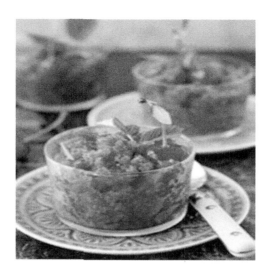

Servings: 4
Total Prep time: 35 minutes

Ingredients
- 4 cups cherries, pitted + extra for garnishing
- 4 tablespoons cherry syrup
- 3 cups water
- 4 teaspoons vanilla extract
- 4 tablespoons sugar
- 20 ice cubes

Directions
1. Add cherries, water, sugar, and cherry syrup to a heavy bottomed pot.
2. Place the pot over medium heat and simmer until cherries are cooked.
3. When done, cool slightly and blend in a blender.
4. Transfer into a bowl. Add ice cubes to a food processor and pulse until crushed. Transfer crushed into glasses.

5. Pour blended cherry over it.
6. Garnish with cherries and serve immediately.
7. Enjoy!

93)   Strawberry Lemonade Slush

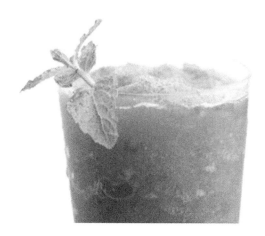

Servings: 8
Total Prep time: 22 minutes

Ingredients
- 1 cup fresh strawberries, chopped roughly
- Zest of 1/2 lemon
- Juice of 1 lemon
- 2-3 tablespoons sugar or to taste
- 1 1/2 cups water
- 1 cup ice cubes

Directions
1. Add all the ingredients except ice to a blender and blend until smooth.
2. Add in the ice cubes and blend until it gets slush like texture.
3. Pour into 2 tall glasses and serve immediately. Enjoy!

94)   Pinacolada Ice

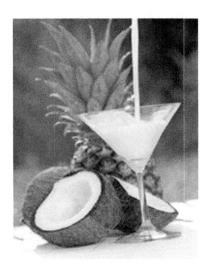

Servings: 8
Total Prep time: 5 minutes

Ingredients

- 1 cup canned pineapple juice
- 2 frozen bananas, chopped
- 4 cups fresh pineapple pieces
- 1 cup coconut milk
- 2 cups crushed ice

Directions

1. Add all the ingredients except ice to a blender and blend until smooth.
2. Finally, add in the ice cubes and blend until it gets slush like texture.
3. Serve immediately.
4. Enjoy!

95)   Fruit Ice

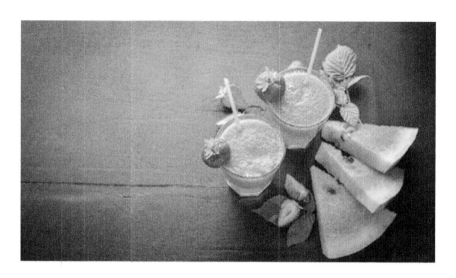

Servings: 2
Total Prep time: 5 minutes

Ingredients
- 1 cup fruit juice of your choice
- 2 cups crushed ice

Directions
1. Add juice ice to a blender and blend until it gets a slush like texture
2. Serve immediately.
3. Enjoy!

96) Orange Frozen Yogurt

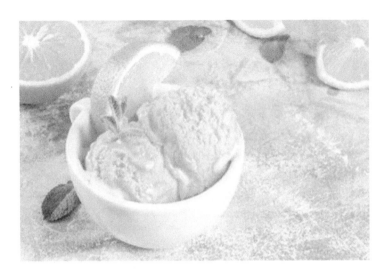

Servings: 8
Total Prep time: 3 hours 1 0 minutes

Ingredients:
- 2 Cups Blood Orange Juice
- 2 Cups Greek Yogurt
- 1 Tbsp Blood Orange Zest
- 1/3 Cup Date Syrup
- 1 Tsp Vanilla Essence

Directions
1. In a bowl whisk together the blood orange juice and yogurt until well mixed and smooth and creamy in consistency
2. Add the date syrup and vanilla essence and mix thoroughly until well combined
3. Pour into Popsicle molds and freeze for 3 hours.

97)   Banana Chip Frozen Yogurt

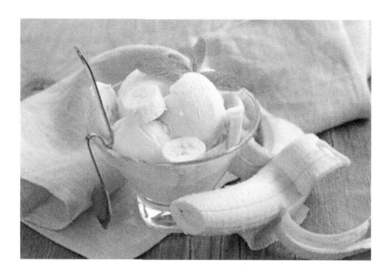

Servings: 6
Total Prep time: 4 hours 20 minutes

Ingredients:
- 4 Ripe Bananas, peeled
- 2 Cups Greek Yogurt
- 1 Cup Condensed Milk
- A Large Handful of Banana Chips

Directions
1. Puree the bananas, yogurt, and milk in a blender until silky in consistency and pour into a plastic container
2. Place the banana chips in a bag and bash with a rolling pin to make banana crumbs. Sprinkle the crumbs on top of the yogurt mixture.
3. Cover and freeze for at least 4 hours

98) Rum and Raisin Frozen Yogurt

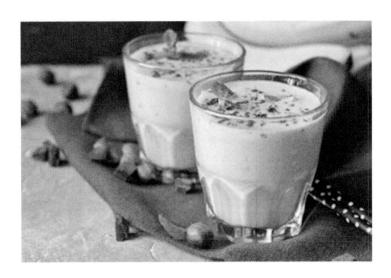

Servings: 8
Total Prep time: 12 hours 20 minutes

Ingredients:
- 3 Cups Coconut Yogurt
- 2/3 Cup Sugar
- 2/3 Cup Raisins
- 2 Tbsps. Dark Rum
- 2 Tsps. Vanilla Extract
- A Pinch of Salt

Directions
1. Put the coconut yogurt in a strainer lined with cheesecloth and place over a pot.
2. Leave in the fridge for at least 8 hours until all the water has drained out of the yogurt. Mix the strained yogurt with the sugar, raisins, rum, vanilla, and salt until well combined.

3. Cover and place in the fridge overnight to allow the flavors to develop.
4. Place the mixture in an ice cream maker and follow the instructions for frozen yogurt and then freeze for 4 hours.
5. Enjoy.

99)   Chai Frozen Yogurt

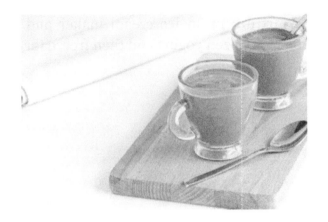

Servings: 4
Total Prep time: 4 hours 15 minutes

Ingredients:
- 2 Chai Teabags
- 3/4 Cups Water
- 32oz Vanilla Greek Yogurt
- Pinch of Cinnamon
- Pinch of Cardamom
- Pinch of Ground Ginger
- 1 Tbsp Sugar

Directions
1. Put the chai tea bags in boiling water and then leave to cool completely
2. Mix all the ingredients in a bowl and add the cooled tea
3. Place in an ice cream maker and follow the instructions for frozen yogurt
4. Put in the freezer for 4 hours or eat immediately if you prefer a softer consistency

100) Blackberry and Lavender Frozen Yogurt Popsicles

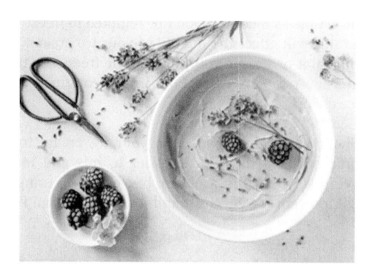

Servings: 6
Total Prep time: 5 hours 20 minutes

Ingredients:
- 13oz Greek Yogurt
- 3/4 Cup Milk
- 4 Tbsps. Blackberry Jam
- 2 Punnets Fresh Blackberries 1
- Tbsp Vanilla Extract
- 1 Tsp Dried Lavender

Directions
1. Put the yogurt, milk, jam, blackberries, and vanilla in a blender and blend until smooth. Add the lavender and pulse to combine.
2. Pour into molds and freeze for 5 hours before serving.

TIPS AND TRICKS

1. Pre-freeze your bowl for 24 hours, but it can also be as little time as 8 hours. Don't be tempted to freeze for less as this will affect the quality of your ice cream. Get in the habit of storing your bowl in the freezer so that you are never caught short. Cold ingredients make quicker ice cream.

2. Shallow containers will help your ice cream to freeze quicker and will make it easier to mix and to scoop. Wrap your bowl in a plastic bag before freezing. This will prevent freezer burn and ice crystals from building up.

3. Make the mixture in advance and keep the mix in the fridge overnight to quicken the process with an ice cream making method.

4. Use the freshest ingredients available and those in 'season' and no preservatives, additives, etc. For the best flavor. Homemade ice cream uses fresh ingredients, so you should try and eat it within a week, or it will begin to lose flavor. Don't store your ice cream for too long. It will lose some of its flavor and texture over time, and the lack of preservatives present in shop bought ice cream means it's best to eat as quickly as possible – ideally within a week or two weeks maximum.

5. If you substitute ingredients for low-fat alternatives, you will save some calories, but the ice cream will not taste as good.

6. With any recipe that calls for egg yolks, if you add hot liquid too quickly to the eggs, they will scramble, and that is almost the opposite of ice cream.

7. If you want to mix any additional ingredients into your ice creams, such as nuts, dried fruits, chocolate chips or chunks of peanut brittle, add them in the right at the end of the process for the best results

8. Alcohol can be fun (for adults, definitely not for kids), but more alcohol means more time to freeze, or your ice cream not freezing at all. Use alcohol to flavor, not to booze your ice cream up.

9. All recipes are best eaten immediately, however, if you do wish to freeze them store your ice cream, yogurts or sorbets in flat plastic containers in the freezer. This will allow for more even consistency.

10. To prevent ice crystals from forming on the top of ice cream place a layer of cling film or greaseproof paper over the top before putting on the lid.

11. Do not refreeze ice cream that has thawed as this will pose a risk of bacteria growing.

12. Do not overfill the bowl. Three-quarters full should be the maximum to allow air to get into the mixture.

13. To serve ice cream that has been frozen, remove from the freezer 10 minutes before serving or to the refrigerator for 30 minutes.

14. To scoop ice cream perfectly from the container using a spring-loaded scoop dipped in warm water.

CONCLUSION

Well, what a journey we have been on. I hope that you and your loved ones will enjoy making these yummy homemade ice cream recipes. As far as I know, ice cream is not seen as a health food, or is it? No, it most definitely is not. It is yummy though! I can assure you that you will feel so much better offering your loved ones these sweet, cold treats especially over the summer.

Once you have mastered ice cream making, you will never buy ice cream from a store again. Try out the recipes and see what works for you. Do not be afraid to experiment and try new things. Find out what you like and what you don't like and make some great ice cream. Some of the methods and recipes take no time at all, while some take all the time in the world if you do this right, you will be feeding your heart and soul, as well as the hearts and souls around you.

I wish to thank you once again for downloading my book; your support of my work is very much appreciated. Good luck on your journey to the land of sweet treats and frozen goodness. Pick up your spoon, thrust it in the air and claim your spot as a hero for the ages!

Printed in Great Britain
by Amazon